Diagnosis and Management of Pediatric Diseases

Diagnosis and Management of Pediatric Diseases

Special Issue Editor

Consolato M. Sergi

MDPI • Basel • Beijing • Wuhan • Barcelona • Belgrade

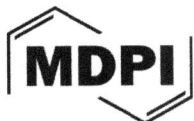

MDPI

Special Issue Editor
Consolato M. Sergi
University of Alberta, Edmonton
Canada

Editorial Office
MDPI
St. Alban-Anlage 66
4052 Basel, Switzerland

This is a reprint of articles from the Special Issue published online in the open access journal *Diagnostics* (ISSN 2075-4418) from 2018 to 2019 (available at: https://www.mdpi.com/journal/diagnostics/special_issues/Pediatric).

For citation purposes, cite each article independently as indicated on the article page online and as indicated below:

LastName, A.A.; LastName, B.B.; LastName, C.C. Article Title. *Journal Name* **Year**, *Article Number*, Page Range.

ISBN 978-3-03921-966-7 (Pbk)
ISBN 978-3-03921-967-4 (PDF)

Cover image courtesy of Consolato M. Sergi.

Contents

About the Special Issue Editor

Consolato M. Sergi, MD, Ph.D., FRCPC, FCAP is Full Professor of Pathology and Adjunct Professor at the Department of Pediatrics, University of Alberta, Edmonton, Canada. Dr. Sergi holds two specializations (Pediatrics and Pathology) and a fellowship in Pediatric Pathology. Dr. Sergi is Fellow of the Royal College of Physicians and Surgeons of Canada and Fellow of the College of the American Pathologists. Dr. Sergi's interests are congenital heart disease and metabolic diseases, biliary diseases of the liver (intra- and extrahepatic), carcinogenesis (bone/soft tissue/liver), and cardiomyopathies of youth. Dr. Sergi has more than 250 peer-reviewed PubMed publications. Dr. Sergi sits on the board of IARC/WHO, involved in the revision of chemical compounds as well as reviewing the guidelines for carcinogenesis in experimental animal models linked to several chemical compounds of public interest. Dr. Sergi is a member of numerous medical professional societies and is a member of the editorial board of numerous prestigious medical journals.

diagnostics

MDPI

Editorial

Pediatrics: An Evolving Concept for the 21st Century

Consolato M. Sergi [1,2]

[1]   Stollery Children's Hospital, Department of Laboratory Medicine and Pathology, University of Alberta, Edmonton, AB T6G 2B7, Canada; sergi@ualberta.ca
[2]   National "111" Center for Cellular Regulation and Molecular Pharmaceutics, Hubei University of Technology, Wuhan 430068, China

Received: 20 November 2019; Accepted: 20 November 2019; Published: 25 November 2019

Pediatrics is rapidly evolving, and the diagnostic tools are expanding the spectrum of diagnoses that can be identified at the bedside. The recent progress identified in pediatrics of the last 20 years is astonishing and has consolidated the concept that children are not "smaller adults" and indeed, perinatal and pediatric pathology has become an independent subspecialty in pathology with impressive intersections with fetal medicine, neonatology, and pediatrics. The neonatal intensive care unit (NICU) as well as the pediatric intensive care unit (PICU) play a major role in modern hospitals. These sections of the hospital provide sick newborns and children with the highest level of medical care. Differently from the general medical floors, both units allow intensive nursing care and continuous monitoring of vital parameters, including heart rate, breathing, and blood pressure. The survival of premature babies and small for date newborns has increased exponentially in the last few decades. On the other hand, the immune system, as well as the pulmonary and gastrointestinal organs, remain difficult to manage. At this age an increased rate of infection has been identified, and gastrointestinal dysfunction is common [1–6]. Cardiovascular function and sepsis are intimately related and may trigger early death without NICU or PICU intervention [7]. Although the diagnostic procedures in newborns are often overlapping with diagnostic algorithms used at older age, they continue to be a complex and dynamic process which requires a proper investigation of the obstetrical and medical history, skillful physical examination, appropriate laboratory tests, and imaging studies with or without pathological examination of tissue biopsies. On the other hand, even with these steps, diagnosis may remain elusive. The journey from the first appearance of symptom or sign to the final diagnosis may seem sometimes interminable. Today, new techniques seem to shorten this journey swiftly, and next-generation sequencing (NGS) will play a major role in the next decade. NGS is becoming more and more used in clinics other than in academia, although one of the most challenging aspects of NGS testing may reside in its analytical validity. The field of metabolomics is indeed developing at a remarkable rate, particularly in pediatrics. Over the last few years, the pre-clinical detection of pathologies has become more robust and efficient. In electronic libraries, new biomarkers are being identified for several pathologies in neonatology and pediatrics. Management of pediatric diseases may become extenuating, and the use of single nucleotide polymorphisms for the improvement of our approach to some pediatric diagnostic algorithmic failures targeting the interindividual variability may be considered. Pediatric trial networks provide pediatricians, researchers, and agencies with new information on how children may respond to drugs and medications. The present Special Issue collects wet lab research and review articles to highlight some fields of pediatrics that may shape future directions in the diagnosis and management of some diseases. Pediatric heart failure is a challenge in neonatology and pediatrics, and quality assurance criteria are key [7–11]. An open-heart surgery with cardiopulmonary bypass (CPB) remains an interventional procedure accompanied by a high mortality/morbidity rate. Satriano et al. investigated whether blood concentrations of glutathione (GSH), a powerful endogenous antioxidant, changed in the perioperative period [12]. In the perioperative period, the increase in GSH may suggest that a compensatory mechanism to oxidative damage during surgical procedure takes place. The measurement of the interferon (IFN) score has been suggested for the screening of monogenic interferonopathies, like the Aicardi–Goutières syndrome. Moreover, it may be useful to stratify subjects with systemic lupus erythematosus before receiving IFN-targeted treatments. Pin et al. developed an approach to reduce the inter-laboratory variability [13]. These authors provide shared strategies for the IFN signature analysis. They allow different centers to compare data and merge their experiences. Diabetic retinopathy (DR) is a dramatic and major microvascular complication of diabetes mellitus, and very few studies have evidenced the magnitude of this disorder in the pediatric population [14]. The International Society for Pediatric and Adolescent Diabetes (ISPAD) mandates that annual screening for DR should be performed in patients aged 11 years after diabetes of 2 years' duration and from 9 years of age with diabetes of 5 years' duration [15]. Kołodziej et al. studied the width of individual retinal layers in patients with type 1 diabetes (T1DM) correlating their data with markers of diabetes metabolic control applying the optical coherence tomography (OCT) study performed using a high definition OCT Cirrus 5000 [16]. The authors found a positive correlation between center thickness and spectral-domain for average glycemia and temporal CT with age at examination, suggesting that selected parameters may be applied as potential markers of preclinical phase of DR in patients with T1DM. Allen and Gupta highlight the current and nearest futuristic perspective of "artificial pancreas" suggesting that soon such a system may not require any manual patient input allowing patients to eat throughout the day without entering any blood sugars or counting carbohydrates [17]. Such a device may be commercially available as technology continues to advance in this direction using artificial intelligence. Sarcoidosis is an inflammatory syndrome of non-necrotizing granulomatous type with multisystemic manifestations, and its occurrence in pediatrics is not an isolated finding any longer. Few cases have been reported of this intriguing disease in children and youth [18]. Chiu et al. revised this topic in detail in this issue [19]. These authors focused on early-onset sarcoidosis, high-risk sarcoidosis, and atypical sarcoid-related diseases. Blau syndrome and early-onset sarcoidosis occur in children younger than five years manifesting with extra-thoracic findings but usually without lymphadenopathy and pulmonary involvement. Endoscopic bronchial ultrasound (EBUS) and transbronchial fine-needle aspiration (TBNA) sampling of intrathoracic lymph nodes and lung may provide good diagnostic yield and excellent patient safety profile in childhood. Respiratory syncytial virus (RSV) bronchiolitis remains an important cause of morbidity in early infancy. RSV belongs to the species of *Orthopneumovirus*. The human RSV (HRSV) infects 60% of infants during their first RSV season, and usually all children show an infection record with this virus by 2–3 years of age [20]. Among the infants infected with RSV, 2–3% will develop bronchiolitis, necessitating hospitalization [21]. RSV bronchiolitis is a major cause of infection and hospitalization in infancy and childhood worldwide. Palivizumab can be employed to prevent this infection in preterm babies, infants with certain congenital heart defects (CHD), infants affected with bronchopulmonary dysplasia (BPD), and infants with congenital malformations of the airway. HRSV bronchiolitis is treated with supportive care, including oxygen therapy, continuous positive airway pressure (CPAP) or nasal high flow oxygen, as required. Rodriguez-Gonzalez et al. identified that left ventricular myocardial dysfunction (LVMD) might occur in healthy infants with HRSV bronchiolitis who develop severe disease and need to be treated at the PICU [22]. N-terminal pro-B-type natriuretic peptide (NT-proBNP) seems to increase the accuracy of traditional clinical markers in predicting the outcomes. Duvekot et al. report a rare event complicating a common adenotonsillectomy. Subcutaneous and mediastinal emphysema followed by group A beta-hemolytic streptococci mediastinitis occurred in a young child, reminding us the life-threatening complications of such surgical procedure [23]. Primary indications for adenotonsillectomy are obstructive sleep apnea (OSA) and recurrent pharyngotonsillitis. Although there is evidence-based medicine supporting the use of such surgical procedures on children affected with OSA that is mainly derived on sleep studies, quality of life, and child behavior, it seems that the impact of surgery on recurrent sore throat symptoms is less well delineated. It has been indicated that children younger than three years and children with OSA of moderate to severe degree, as well as infants affected with significant comorbidities should be admitted for overnight observation. In most patients, simple analgesia is adequate postoperatively, while codeine is contraindicated due to cases of postoperative death as consequence of respiratory suppression. Pain and postoperative hemorrhage (2–4%) are the most common complications, but bleeding can be life-threatening, nevertheless the mortality rate remains small but substantial (1:30,000) [24]. Besides tonsillar enlargement, salivary gland enlargement is a condition which enters in the differential diagnosis of head and neck (H&N) masses. Branchial cysts, sialadenosis, and inflammation of the salivary glands are often seen in childhood and youth, but H&N malignant pathologies also need to be taken into consideration. Sergi et al. critically review the diagnostic features of a pediatric mass of the H&N region [25]. Somatosensory evoked potentials (SSEPs) are crucial in assessing the functional integrity of the neural pathways and for predicting the outcome of perinatal injuries. Barkhuizen et al. studied the translational potential of SSEPs together with sensory function in rodents with perinatal hypoxic-ischemic events [26]. No group differences in the amplitude or latency of the evoked potentials of the preceding sensory response were seen, but nevertheless this method of study is intriguing for the functional recovery. Das and van Landeghem revise the clinicopathological spectrum of bilirubin encephalopathy/kernicterus, which is relatively rare but continues to occur despite universal newborn screening, particularly in middle and low income countries [27]. The authors illustrate the array of clinicopathological findings, and the procedures of diagnostic testing reported to be key in the context of bilirubin encephalopathy and kernicterus. Khan and Sergi report on sialidosis, which is a rare, autosomal recessive inherited disorder, caused by α-N-acetyl neuraminidase deficiency resulting from a mutation in the neuraminidase gene (*NEU1*) and accompanied by cerebral and extra-cerebral manifestations combining the underlying molecular biology, the clinical features, and the morphological patterns of this disorder [28].

Finally, the attention should be drawn to the frontispiece of this book. It is a photograph of a famous sculpture of Horatio Greenough (6 September 1805–18 December 1852). He was an American sculptor who was best known for his two United States government commissions, "The Rescue" and "George Washington", among others. Before graduating from Harvard, Horatio Greenough sailed to Italy, Rome, to study art. There, the sculptor created many busts. In 1833, he realized "The Ascension of a Child Conducted by an Infant Angel" in marble. The gift to the Museum of Fine Arts in Boston, Massachusetts, United States of America, is a marvelous and touching piece of art and may combine the most elysian characteristics of all Greenough's sculpture. Both the child and the angel are animated by a deep serenity, which may deeply contrast to the austere Hadrian's words engraved in the sculpture support (*Animula, vagula, blandula - Hospes comesque corporis - Quae nunc abibis in loca Pallidula, rigida, nudula - Nec, ut soles, dabis iocos?* Little, suave, and wanderer soul, guest and partner of the body - Where are you off to now? Somewhere without color, severe, and empty - Never will you participate in gags as usual). Publius Aelius Hadrianus Augustus was a Roman emperor from 117 to 138 A.D., who died at the age of 62 years following a long and restless reign. Suffering from hypertension and coronary atherosclerosis in the last years of his life, he probably died of congestive heart failure as extensively reported by Dio Cassius and the Historia Augusta records [29]. This suffering has probably shaped some of his scripts. The "Ascension of a Child Conducted by an Infant Angel" conveys an astonishingly gentle, warm, and attractive message of peacefulness, hope, and spirituality in an age of high infant mortality. In 1911, Newmayer wrote that the country which first recognizes its responsibilities to the child would be given the appreciation of the world as being the leading civilized nation [30]. At this time, the United States lagged in the child's health and welfare, and the infant mortality rate (IMR) positioned the United States as ranked in the 18th position out of 30 countries, with a rate of 135 deaths per 1000 live births. Following the European example, US public health leaders started a national campaign to reduce infant mortality, and, in 1912, the US Children's Bureau (USCB) was founded (Brosco 1999). Federal and state programs multiplied and, progressively, pediatricians and children's hospitals also surfaced as the ideal supply of healthcare for children. The improvement of nutrition and treatment of rickets were also crucial and the results of these efforts during the last century have been impressive in all states consolidating the concept of pediatric healthcare in other countries, such as Canada, as well [31]. Digitalization of the imaging in radiology and pathology is a reality in several healthcare institutions worldwide [32,33]. Advances in medical diagnosis and therapy with the implementation of new technologies will be the basis for the future of pediatric healthcare, personalized pediatrics, and quality assurance and controls in the 21st century.

Conflicts of Interest: The author declares no conflict of interest.

References

1. Sergi, C.; Hager, T.; Hager, J. Congenital Segmental Intestinal Dilatation: A 25-Year Review with Long-Term Follow-up at the Medical University of Innsbruck, Austria. *AJP Rep.* **2019**, *9*, e218–e225. [CrossRef] [PubMed]
2. Sergi, C.M.; Caluseriu, O.; McColl, H.; Eisenstat, D.D. Hirschsprung's disease: Clinical dysmorphology, genes, micro-RNAs, and future perspectives. *Pediatr. Res.* **2017**, *81*, 177–191. [CrossRef] [PubMed]
3. Takawira, C.; D'Agostini, S.; Shenouda, S.; Persad, R.; Sergi, C. Laboratory procedures update on Hirschsprung disease. *J. Pediatr. Gastroenterol. Nutr.* **2015**, *60*, 598–605. [CrossRef] [PubMed]
4. Pelletier, J.S.; LaBossiere, J.; Dicken, B.; Gill, R.S.; Sergi, C.; Tahbaz, N.; Bigam, D.; Cheung, P.Y. Low-dose vasopressin improves cardiac function in newborn piglets with acute hypoxia-reoxygenation. *Shock* **2013**, *40*, 320–326. [CrossRef]
5. Cheung, D.C.; Gill, R.S.; Liu, J.Q.; Manouchehri, N.; Sergi, C.; Bigam, D.; Cheung, P.Y.; Dicken, B.J. Vasopressin improves systemic hemodynamics without compromising mesenteric perfusion in the resuscitation of asphyxiated newborn piglets: A dose-response study. *Intensive Care Med.* **2012**, *38*, 491–498. [CrossRef]
6. Dicken, B.J.; Sergi, C.; Rescorla, F.J.; Breckler, F.; Sigalet, D. Medical management of motility disorders in patients with intestinal failure: A focus on necrotizing enterocolitis, gastroschisis, and intestinal atresia. *J. Pediatr. Surg.* **2011**, *46*, 1618–1630. [CrossRef]
7. Sergi, C.; Shen, F.; Lim, D.W.; Liu, W.; Zhang, M.; Chiu, B.; Anand, V.; Sun, Z. Cardiovascular dysfunction in sepsis at the dawn of emerging mediators. *Biomed. Pharmacother.* **2017**, *95*, 153–160. [CrossRef]
8. Sergi, C.M. Sudden cardiac death and ethnicity. *CMAJ* **2019**, *191*, E1254. [CrossRef]
9. Sergi, C. Customer Care in Pediatric Cardiac Transplant Pathology: Basic Concepts and Critical Analysis in the Setting of Precision Medicine. *Ann. Clin. Lab. Sci.* **2019**, *49*, 682–685.
10. Hsu, Y.H.; Yogasundaram, H.; Parajuli, N.; Valtuille, L.; Sergi, C.; Oudit, G.Y. MELAS syndrome and cardiomyopathy: Linking mitochondrial function to heart failure pathogenesis. *Heart Fail. Rev.* **2016**, *21*, 103–116. [CrossRef]
11. Sergi, C. Promptly reporting of critical laboratory values in pediatrics: A work in progress. *World J. Clin. Pediatr.* **2018**, *7*, 105–110. [CrossRef] [PubMed]
12. Satriano, A.; Franchini, S.; Lapergola, G.; Pluchinotta, F.; Anastasia, L.; Baryshnikova, E.; Livolti, G.; Gazzolo, D. Glutathione Blood Concentrations: A Biomarker of Oxidative Damage Protection during Cardiopulmonary Bypass in Children. *Diagnostics* **2019**, *9*, 118. [CrossRef]
13. Pin, A.; Monasta, L.; Taddio, A.; Piscianz, E.; Tommasini, A.; Tesser, A. An Easy and Reliable Strategy for Making Type I Interferon Signature Analysis Comparable among Research Centers. *Diagnostics* **2019**, *9*, 113. [CrossRef] [PubMed]
14. Wang, S.Y.; Andrews, C.A.; Herman, W.H.; Gardner, T.W.; Stein, J.D. Incidence and Risk Factors for Developing Diabetic Retinopathy among Youths with Type 1 or Type 2 Diabetes throughout the United States. *Ophthalmology* **2017**, *124*, 424–430. [CrossRef] [PubMed]
15. Donaghue, K.C.; Wadwa, R.P.; Dimeglio, L.A.; Wong, T.Y.; Chiarelli, F.; Marcovecchio, M.L.; Salem, M.; Raza, J.; Hofman, P.L.; Craig, M.E.; et al. ISPAD Clinical Practice Consensus Guidelines 2014. Microvascular and macrovascular complications in children and adolescents. *Pediatr. Diabetes* **2014**, *15*, 257–269. [CrossRef]
16. Kolodziej, M.; Waszczykowska, A.; Korzeniewska-Dyl, I.; Pyziak-Skupien, A.; Walczak, K.; Moczulski, D.; Jurowski, P.; Mlynarski, W.; Szadkowska, A.; Zmyslowska, A. The HD-OCT Study May Be Useful in Searching for Markers of Preclinical Stage of Diabetic Retinopathy in Patients with Type 1 Diabetes. *Diagnostics* **2019**, *9*, 105. [CrossRef]
17. Allen, N.; Gupta, A. Current Diabetes Technology: Striving for the Artificial Pancreas. *Diagnostics* **2019**, *9*, 31. [CrossRef]

18. Brunner, J.; Sergi, C.; Muller, T.; Gassner, I.; Prufer, F.; Zimmerhackl, L.B. Juvenile sarcoidosis presenting as Crohn's disease. *Eur. J. Pediatr.* **2006**, *165*, 398–401. [CrossRef]

19. Chiu, B.; Chan, J.; Das, S.; Alshamma, Z.; Sergi, C. Pediatric Sarcoidosis: A Review with Emphasis on Early Onset and High-Risk Sarcoidosis and Diagnostic Challenges. *Diagnostics* **2019**, *9*, 160. [CrossRef]

20. Glezen, W.P.; Taber, L.H.; Frank, A.L.; Kasel, J.A. Risk of primary infection and reinfection with respiratory syncytial virus. *Am. J. Dis. Child.* **1986**, *140*, 543–546. [CrossRef]

21. Hall, C.B.; Weinberg, G.A.; Iwane, M.K.; Blumkin, A.K.; Edwards, K.M.; Staat, M.A.; Auinger, P.; Griffin, M.R.; Poehling, K.A.; Erdman, D.; et al. The burden of respiratory syncytial virus infection in young children. *N. Engl. J. Med.* **2009**, *360*, 588–598. [CrossRef] [PubMed]

22. Rodriguez-Gonzalez, M.; Perez-Reviriego, A.A.; Castellano-Martinez, A.; Lubian-Lopez, S.; Benavente-Fernandez, I. Left Ventricular Dysfunction and Plasmatic NT-proBNP Are Associated with Adverse Evolution in Respiratory Syncytial Virus Bronchiolitis. *Diagnostics* **2019**, *9*, 85. [CrossRef] [PubMed]

23. Duvekot, A.; van Heesch, G.; Veder, L. Subcutaneous and Mediastinal Emphysema Followed by Group A Beta-Hemolytic Streptococci Mediastinitis. A Complicated Course after Adenotonsillectomy: Case Report. *Diagnostics* **2019**, *9*, 11. [CrossRef] [PubMed]

24. Greig, S.R. Current perspectives on the role of tonsillectomy. *J. Paediatr. Child. Health* **2017**, *53*, 1065–1070. [CrossRef]

25. Sergi, C.; Dhiman, A.; Gray, J.A. Fine Needle Aspiration Cytology for Neck Masses in Childhood. An Illustrative Approach. *Diagnostics* **2018**, *8*, 28. [CrossRef]

26. Barkhuizen, M.; Vles, J.S.H.; van Mechelen, R.; Vermeer, M.; Kramer, B.W.; Chedraui, P.; Bergs, P.; van Kranen-Mastenbroek, V.; Gavilanes, A.W.D. Preterm Perinatal Hypoxia-Ischemia Does not Affect Somatosensory Evoked Potentials in Adult Rats. *Diagnostics* **2019**, *9*, 123. [CrossRef]

27. Das, S.; van Landeghem, F.K.H. Clinicopathological Spectrum of Bilirubin Encephalopathy/Kernicterus. *Diagnostics* **2019**, *9*, 24. [CrossRef]

28. Khan, A.; Sergi, C. Sialidosis: A Review of Morphology and Molecular Biology of a Rare Pediatric Disorder. *Diagnostics* **2018**, *8*, 29. [CrossRef]

29. Birley, A. *Hadrian: The Restless Emperor*; Psychology Press: London, UK, 1997.

30. Newmayer, S.W. The warfare against infant mortality. *Ann. Am. Acad. Political Soc. Sci.* **1911**, *37*, 532–542. [CrossRef]

31. Zhang, M.; Shen, F.; Petryk, A.; Tang, J.; Chen, X.; Sergi, C. "English Disease": Historical Notes on Rickets, the Bone-Lung Link and Child Neglect Issues. *Nutrients* **2016**, *8*, 722. [CrossRef]

32. Sergi, C.M. Digital Pathology: The Time Is Now to Bridge the Gap between Medicine and Technological Singularity. In *Interactive Multimedia-Multimedia Production and Digital Storytelling*; Cvetković, D., Ed.; IntechOpen: London, UK, 2019. [CrossRef]

33. Solez, K.; Bernier, A.; Crichton, J.; Graves, H.; Kuttikat, P.; Lockwood, R.; Marovitz, W.F.; Monroe, D.; Pallen, M.; Pandya, S.; et al. Bridging the gap between the technological singularity and mainstream medicine: Highlighting a course on technology and the future of medicine. *Glob. J. Health Sci.* **2013**, *5*, 112–125. [CrossRef] [PubMed]

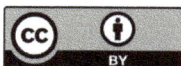

diagnostics

MDPI

Article

Glutathione Blood Concentrations: A Biomarker of Oxidative Damage Protection during Cardiopulmonary Bypass in Children

Angela Satriano [1], Simone Franchini [2], Giuseppe Lapergola [2], Francesca Pluchinotta [1], Luigi Anastasia [1], Ekaterina Baryshnikova [1], Giovanni Livolti [3] and Diego Gazzolo [2,4,*]

[1] Department of Pediatric Cardiac Surgery, IRCCS San Donato Milanese Hospital, San Donato Milanese, 20097 Milan, Italy
[2] Neonatal Intensive Care Unit, G. d'Annunzio University of Chieti, 65100 Chieti, Italy
[3] Department of Biomedical and Biotechnological Sciences Section of Biochemistry University of Catania, 95100 Catania, Italy
[4] AO SS Antonio, Biagio and C. Arrigo Hospital Alessandria, 15121 Alessandria, Italy
* Correspondence: dgazzolo@hotmail.com; Tel.: +39-0131-207241 or +39-0131-207268

Received: 24 July 2019; Accepted: 10 September 2019; Published: 13 September 2019

Abstract: Background. Pediatric open-heart surgery with cardiopulmonary bypass (CPB) still remains a risky interventional procedure at high mortality/morbidity. To date, there are no clinical, laboratory, and/or monitoring parameters providing useful information on perioperative stress. We therefore investigated whether blood concentrations of glutathione (GSH), a powerful endogenous antioxidant, changed in the perioperative period. Methods. We conducted an observational study in 35 congenital heart disease (CHD) children in whom perioperative standard laboratory and monitoring parameters and GSH blood levels were assessed at five monitoring time points. Results. GSH showed a pattern characterized by a progressive increase from pre-surgery up to 24 h after surgery, reaching its highest peak at the end of CPB. GSH measured at the end of CPB correlated with CPB duration, cross-clamping, arterial oxygen partial pressure, and with body core temperature. Conclusions. The increase in GSH levels in the perioperative period suggests a compensatory mechanism to oxidative damage during surgical procedure. Caution is needed in controlling different CPB phases, especially systemic reoxygenation in a population that is per se more prone to oxidative stress/damage. The findings may point the way to detecting the optimal temperature and oxygenation target by biomarker monitoring.

Keywords: GSH; cardiopulmonary bypass; newborn; brain damage; oxidative stress

---

1. Introduction

Pediatric open-heart surgery with cardiopulmonary bypass (CPB) still remains a risky interventional procedure at high mortality and morbidity [1]. Hemodynamic and thermal changes occurring during CPB are known to trigger a cascade of events (i.e., ischemia-reperfusion injury, surgical procedure, endothelial dysfunction, activation of complement, coagulation, and inflammatory processes) that can lead to tissue damage [2].

The assessment of proinflammatory cytokines and intracellular biomarkers has been recently proposed in order to offer useful information on tissue stress in the perioperative period [3]. In this regard, it has been shown that glutathione (GSH) is essential for vascular and cardiac function and determines cell survival [4–7]. Moreover, in humans and in animal heart failure models, exacerbated tumor necrosis factor and soluble tumor necrosis factor receptor-1 expression was related to systemic and cardiac GSH deficiency supporting the notion of GSH's role in the defense against oxidative stress [4,5,8–10].

GSH has been detected in different biological fluids and it has been suggested that its presence provides a good source of this protective antioxidant for newborns. GSH performs several important physiological functions, such as (a) inactivation of oxygen-derived highly reactive species [10,11]; (b) detoxification of various types of xenobiotics and carcinogens [10,12]; (c) maintenance of the oxidative status of other antioxidants, such as ascorbic acid and α-tocopherol [13]; and (d) cell immune response improvement by activation of lymphocytes [14]. In this light, GSH in adults undergoing surgical repair with CPB has been shown to increase, reflecting a cellular defense mechanism against oxidative damage during reperfusion [15]. Conversely, data on GSH concentrations in children, affected by congenital heart disease (CHD) and undergoing cardiac surgery, are still lacking or are a matter of debate. Reduced GSH levels has been recently shown to play an important role in inflammatory response [3], whereas changes in GSH blood levels were observed according to different CPB phases (i.e., controlled anterograde low oxygen warm reperfusion before de-clamping and aortic cross-clamping release) [15].

Therefore, in the present observational study we investigated whether, in CHD children undergoing cardiac surgery with CPB, blood concentrations of a powerful endogenous antioxidant, namely GSH, changed in the perioperative period.

2. Materials and Methods

We conducted an observational study at our third-level referral center for pediatric cardiac diseases of 35 CHD children without pre-existing neurological disorders or other co-morbidities. CHD characteristics as well as main interventions and clinical laboratory parameters recorded at admission into the study are reported in Table 1.

Table 1. Laboratory parameters, main interventions, and general characteristics of the children with complications of congenital heart disease (CHD) admitted into the study.

	CHD (*n* = 35)
CHD characteristics	
Tetralogy of Fallot	15
Transposition of great arteries	6
Tricuspid atresia	8
Total anomalous pulmonary venous return	6
Age (months)	30 ± 8
Weight (kg)	11 ± 2
Gender (F/M)	10/25
Laboratory parameters	
Hemoglobin (g/dL)	12.3 ± 1.2
Hematocrit (%)	35.5 ± 2.9
Platelet count (10^3/mmc)	325 ± 102
Creatinine (mg/dL)	0.43 ± 0.25
Urea (mg/dL)	29 ± 14
LDH (UI/L)	565 ± 206
CK (UI/L)	168 ± 114
Glycaemia (mg/dL)	103 ± 12
Neurological examination	
Preoperative (normal/suspect/abnormal)	35/0/0
Postoperative (normal/suspect/abnormal)	35/0/0
Main interventions	
CPB (min)	90 ± 66
Filtration (*n*/total)	19/25
Clamping (min)	46 ± 34
Circulatory arrest (*n*/total)	2/25
Cooling (°C)	31.9 ± 3.1

Abbreviations: LDH, lactate dehydrogenase; CK, creatine kinase, CPB, cardiopulmonary bypass.

Informed and signed consent from parents was obtained, before the patients' inclusion in the study, which was approved by the local human investigation committee (N718, EC Policlinico San Donato Milanese, 12, 12, 2012).

At admission to our unit, all children underwent clinical and standard laboratory and monitoring parameter recordings and GSH assessment. Blood samples were drawn at five predetermined times before, during, and after surgery, namely, before the surgical procedure and anesthesia (time 0, T0); during the surgical procedure after sternotomy and before CPB (time 1, T1); at the end of CPB (time 2, T2); at the end of the surgical procedure (time 3, T3); 24 h after the surgical procedure (time 4, T4). The following parameters were also recorded: peripheral temperature; nasopharyngeal temperature; pump flow rate; heart rate (HR) mean arterial systolic and diastolic blood pressure (BP); left and right atrium BP (LA, RA); pulsed arterial oxygen tension (SaO$_2$); and laboratory parameters such as arterial blood pH and oxygen (PaO$_2$) and carbon dioxide (PaCO$_2$) partial pressures, bicarbonate (HCO$_3$), base excess (BE), and hemoglobin (Hb) concentrations, hematocrit rate (Ht), platelet count, and creatinine, urea, lactate dehydrogenase, creatine kinase, and glucose blood levels.

2.1. Anesthetic Technique

After premedication with midazolam (Ipnovel, Roche, Milan, Italy), 0.5 mg/kg·bw (intramuscular), induction was achieved with oxygen and 3% sevofluorane (SevoFlo, Zoetis Belgium SA, Louvain-la-Neuve, Belgium) administered via mask (single-breath induction), followed by intravenous sufentanil (Fentanest, Pharmacia and Upjohn, Milan, Italy) 1 (g/kg·bw) and vecuronium (Norcuron, NV organon, Oss, The Netherlands) (0.15 mg/kg·bw). Maintenance was achieved with 3% sevofluorane (except during CPB) and with additional doses of sufentanil (0.5 g/kg·bw) and vecuronium (0.1 mg/kg·bw) every 30–40 min. During CPB, in the absence of sevofluorane, additional midazolam at 0.2 mg/kg·bw dosage was given. Sufentanil infusion at 0.25 g/kg·bw was continued in the intensive care unit for sedation [16].

2.2. Cardiopulmonary Bypass Management

The study population underwent a CPB procedure according to our protocols [16]. CPB was established after systemic heparinization (3 mg/kg·bw) by standard single-stage aortic and bicaval cannulation, and maintained via non-pulsatile pump flow with a membrane oxygenator (Dideco Laboratories, Modena, Italy). Flow velocity was kept at 120–150 mL/kg·bw, and mean arterial blood pressure at 45 mmHg; hypothermia was attained by core and surface cooling. Three patients were operated in deep hypothermic circulatory arrest (DHCA) (19 ± 7 min) and the minimum temperature reached was 25 °C. Mean rewarming time was calculated from the final temperature during hypothermic circulatory arrest to 36.5 °C. The pump priming solution was composed of electrolyte solutions (Normosol-R 250 to 650 mL, Abbott Hospital Products, Abbott Park, IL, USA or Plasma-Lyte A, Travenol Laboratories, Inc., Deerfield, IL, USA), albumin (25%), heparin 1000 to 5000 units in the total solution, sodium bicarbonate (25–30 mEq/L), and packed red blood cells or fresh frozen plasma. A standard total circuit prime volume was used, according to body weight, varying from 400 mL (bw < 4.5 kg), to 600 mL (bw > 4.5 kg and bw < 7.5 kg) and to 700 mL (bw > 7.7 kg). Packed red blood cells (200 to 500 mL) were transfused as needed to maintain a hematocrit level above 30% during CPB. Protamine (1 mg for each mg of heparin) was administered at the end of CPB. The α-stat regimen was used, and the PaCO$_2$ maintained between 35 and 40 mmHg, without mathematical correction for the effects of the temperature, by varying the membrane oxygenator gas flow [16].

Modified ultrafiltration (MUF) was routinely performed before removal of arterial and venous cannulae. In the CPB circuit, the arterial line was connected to the inlet and the venous line to the outlet of the ultrafilter. As the patient was separated from the CPB, the clamp was removed from the inlet of the filter, allowing the blood to flow through the arterial line to the filter (10–15 mL/kg/min) and, finally, from a venous line to the RA. The filter allows the passage of molecules smaller than 65 kD molecular weight. When it was necessary to maintain the intravascular volume and stabilize the hemodynamics, the blood returned via the venous reservoir and the venous cannula to the RA. This technique was performed until the Ht achieved the target of 35% [17].

2.3. GSH Measurement

Levels of nonproteic thiol groups were measured in 200 µL of blood, in accordance with the method presented by Hu [18], with partial modifications. This spectrophotometric assay is based on the reaction of thiol groups with 2,2-dithio-bis-nitrobenzoic acid (DTNB) in absolute ethanol to give a colored compound absorbing at $\lambda = 412$ nm. Since the DTNB method is strongly affected by pH, the possibility of avoiding acids (trichloroacetic or sulfosalicylic acid) to precipitate proteins represents a remarkable advantage to ensure the accuracy of the assay. We then carried out the removal of proteins with an excess of absolute ethanol, followed by centrifugation at 3000*g* for 10 min at room temperature. Each value represents the mean ± SD of three experimental determinations for each sample. Results were expressed as micromoles per milliliter of blood.

2.4. Neurological Follow-up

Neurological examination was performed daily according to Prechtl [19]. Each child was assigned to one of three diagnostic groups—normal, suspect, abnormal. A child was considered to be abnormal when one or more of the following neurological syndromes were unequivocally present: (a) increased or decreased excitability (hyperexcitability syndrome, convulsion, apathy syndrome, coma); (b) increased or decreased motility (hyperkinesia, hypokinesia); (c) increased or decreased tonus (hypertonia, hypotonia); (d) asymmetries (peripheral or central); (e) defects of the central nervous system; (f) any combination of the above. When indications of the presence of a syndrome were non-conclusive or if only isolated symptoms were present (e.g., mild hypotonia or only a slight tremor), the children were classified as suspect. Abnormal and suspect cases were excluded from the study.

2.5. Statistical Analysis

For the calculation of sample size, we used GSH changes as the main parameter. As no basic data are available for a studied population, we assumed a decrease of 0.5 SD in GSH to be clinically significant. Indeed, considering $\alpha = 0.05$ and using a two-sided test, we estimated a power of 0.80 recruiting 33 CHD patients. We added $n = 2$ cases to allow any dropout. The sample size was calculated by using nQuery Advisor (Statistical Solutions, Saugus, MA, USA), version 5.0. The Kolmogorov–Smirnov test showed values having a Gaussian distribution, and data were expressed as the mean (SD). Statistical significance was assessed using one-way ANOVA for repeated measures (followed by the post-hoc Tukey test for multiple comparisons) and the unpaired *t*-test when only two groups were compared. Linear regression analysis was used for correlation between GSH and CPB and laboratory parameters. Statistical significance was set at $p < 0.05$.

3. Results

Monitoring and laboratory variables at the predetermined perioperative time points are shown in Table 2. Clinical parameters recorded during surgery remained within limits regarded as within the reference ranges during this type of procedure. No significant differences from T0 to T4 ($p > 0.05$, for all) were observed regarding hemoglobin concentration; hematocrit rate; arterial blood pH, $PaCO_2$, HCO_3, BE, and SaO_2; HR; LA BP; RA BP; systolic and diastolic BP; and glucose blood levels. PaO_2 showed a pattern, from T0 to T4, characterized by a significant ($p < 0.01$, for all) progressive increase in concentration reaching its highest peak at T2 ($p < 0.001$) and progressively decreasing at the end of surgery up to 24 h after the surgical procedure (Table 2).

Table 2. Laboratory parameters at different monitoring time points (before the surgical procedure, T0; during the surgical procedure before CPB, T1; at the end of CPB, T2; at the end of the surgical procedure, T3; 24 h after the surgical procedure, T4) in children admitted into the study. Data are given as mean ± SD.

Parameters	T0	T1	T2	T3	T4
Hemoglobin (g/dL)	11.7 ± 2.2	11.5 ± 2.4	11 ± 2.9	11.1 ± 1.4	11.8 ± 1.5
Hematocrit rate (%)	35.9 ± 3.8	33.8 ± 5.4	32.9 ± 6.3	33.4 ± 4.2	34.5 ± 4.7
pH	7.36 ± 0.10	7.36 ± 0.10	7.38 ± 0.08	7.39 ± 0.08	7.42 ± 0.07
$PaCO_2$ (mmHg)	36.9 ± 6.6	35.4 ± 3.9	34.4 ± 5.5	35.5 ± 5.1	36.2 ± 5.9
PaO_2 (mmHg)	101 ± 37	144 ± 78 *	211 ± 101 *	163 ± 96 *	155 ± 86 *
HCO_3 (mmol/L)	22.1 ± 3.1	22.2 ± 3.9	21.1 ± 3.2	21.2 ± 1.9	22.2 ± 1.8
BE (mmol/L)	0.2 ± 2.5	−1.8 ± 3.6	−3.0 ± 2.1	−0.5 ± 0.7	1.5 ± 1.5
SaO_2 (mmHg)	94.9 ± 8.8	93.8 ± 7.2	97.3 ± 1.8	92.7 ± 2.6	95.3 ± 5.5
Heart rate (bpm)	104 ± 11	113 ± 14	121 ± 14	122 ± 12	125 ± 19
LA BP (mmHg)	8.0 ± 3.9	7.7 ± 4.0	9.2 ± 3.5	9.5 ± 4.2	9.3 ± 4.0
RA BP (mmHg)	9.1 ± 2.2	8.7 ± 1.6	8.8 ± 2.1	9.8 ± 2.3	10 ± 2.8
Systolic BP (mmHg)	88 ± 12	87 ± 17	86 ± 14	95 ± 15	96 ± 13
Diastolic BP (mmHg)	42 ± 11	53 ± 10	54 ± 10	56 ± 10	57 ± 11
Glycaemia (mg/dl)	103 ± 12	118 ± 11	130 ± 19	125 ± 15	119 ± 14

* $p < 0.05$ vs. T0. Abbreviations: arterial carbon dioxide partial pressure, $PaCO_2$; arterial oxygen partial pressure, PaO_2; arterial bicarbonate level, HCO_3; base excess, BE; arterial oxygen saturation, SaO_2; left atrium, LA; blood pressure, BP; right atrium, RA.

No overt neurological injury was observed in surviving patients during the first week after surgery. In CHD children, GSH blood levels were measurable at all monitoring time points. GSH showed a pattern characterized by a progressive increase from T0 (before surgery) to T4 (at 24 h after surgery), reaching its highest peak at T3 (at the end of CPB) and remaining at high levels up to T4 ($p < 0.01$, for all) (Figure 1).

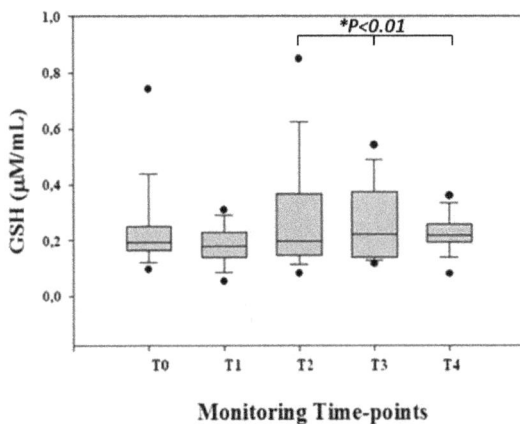

Figure 1. GSH concentrations (μM/mL) expressed as median and 5°–95° centiles at different monitoring time points: before the surgical procedure (T0); during the surgical procedure after sternotomy and before CPB (T1); at the end of CPB (T2); at the end of the surgical procedure (T3); and at 24 h after the surgical procedure (T4) in congenital heart disease children. GSH was significantly (*$p < 0.01$, for all) higher at T3 and T4 vs. T0 monitoring time points.

No significant differences ($p > 0.05$, for both) in GSH levels were shown from T0 to T2. Moreover, in order to evaluate the potential side effects of PaO_2 on GSH levels, we calculated the PaO_2/GSH ratio.

The PaO$_2$/GSH pattern was characterized by a significant ($p < 0.05$, for all) increase from T0 to T3, whereas no differences ($p > 0.05$) were found between T0 and T4.

Linear regression analysis showed a significant correlation between GSH levels measured at the end of CPB (T2). In particular, a positive significant correlation was found with CPB duration (R = 0.72; $p < 0.001$), with cross-clamping (R = 0.62, $p < 0.001$), and with PaO$_2$ (R = 0.53; $p = 0.002$), whereas a negative significant correlation was observed with body core temperature (R = −0.49; $p = 0.012$) (Figures 2–4).

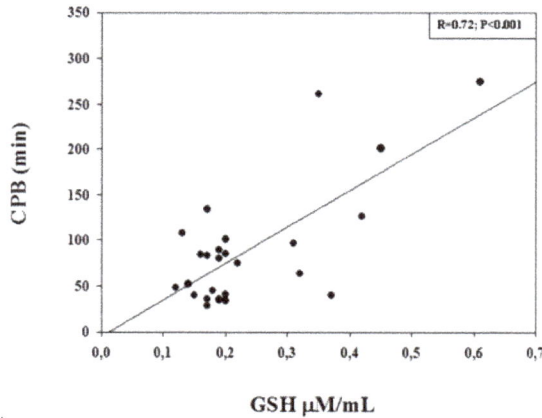

Figure 2. Correlation between GSH concentrations (μM/mL) measured at the end of cardiopulmonary bypass (CPB) procedure and CPB duration (min). There was a significant positive correlation (R = 0.72; $p < 0.001$).

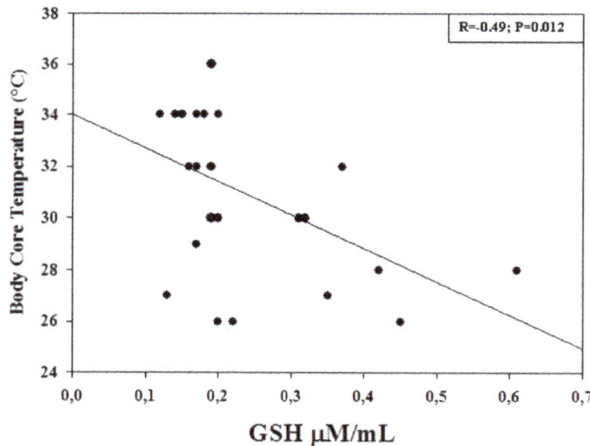

Figure 3. Correlation between GSH concentrations (μM/mL) measured at the end of cardiopulmonary bypass (CPB) procedure and body core temperature (°C) during CPB. There was a significant negative correlation (R = −0.49; $p = 0.012$).

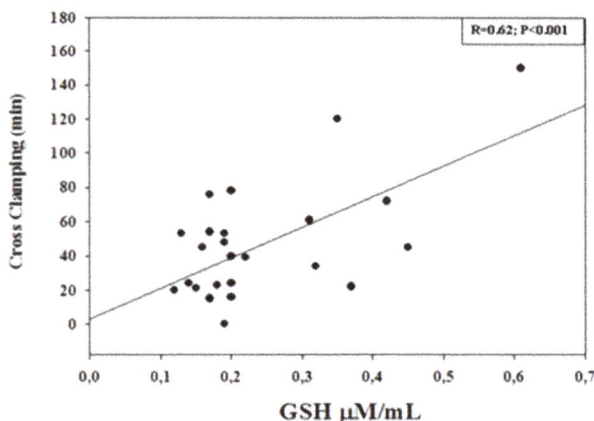

Figure 4. Correlation between GSH concentrations (μM/mL) measured at the end of cardiopulmonary bypass (CPB) procedure and cross-clamping duration (min). There was a significant positive correlation ($R = 0.62$; $p < 0.001$).

Moreover, an identical pattern was found when PaO_2/GSH was correlated with CPB duration ($R = 0.56$; $p = 0.004$), with cross-clamping ($R = 0.51$, $p < 0.010$), and with body core temperature ($R = 0.68$; $p < 0.001$).

4. Discussion

It is widely known that congenital heart diseases are the most frequent malformations, affecting 1–20 infants in 1000 live births [1]. According to CHD characteristics, they may account for up to 15% of mortality, as well as about 4.8% of short-term and 40–50% of long-term developmental abnormalities at school age [1,20,21]. However, there are still no conclusive clinical, laboratory, or monitoring parameters able to provide useful information on perioperative stress [22–25]. In this setting, open-heart surgery and CPB are commonly accepted to cause harmful effects on whole body organs. Vascular resistance impairment, intra/postoperative hypoperfusion leading to ischemia reperfusion injury, and systemic inflammation are known to enhance an oxidative stress reaction in the perioperative period [26].

In the present study, we found that the blood levels of a well-established marker of oxidative stress, namely GSH, significantly increased during surgical procedure by CPB, remaining constantly elevated up to 24 h after surgery. Furthermore, GSH levels measured at the end of the CPB procedure positively correlated with CPB, cross-clamp duration, and PaO_2, whereas a negative correlation was observed with body core temperature. These results are, in part, in agreement with previous observations in adults and in children [15,27], showing increased GSH levels in the postoperative period and in the different CPB phases. Discrepancies are in relation to the different monitoring time points, CPB procedure, and patient recruitment [15].

The finding of elevated GSH levels in the perioperative period warrants further consideration. In particular, increased GSH levels during CPB procedure are (1) related to enhanced oxidative damage due to hypoxia or hyperoxia insults during CPB itself [2]; (2) correlated with the complexity of surgical procedures, especially in those cases requiring DHCA [23]; (3) temperature-dependent due to changes in the oxygen–hemoglobin dissociation curve, enhancing hemoglobin affinity for oxygen with an increase in reduced/oxidized glutathione ratio [28]; and, (4) related to the use of hyperoxic anesthesia that stimulates the production of reactive nitrogen and oxygen species (RNOS) by neutrophils and mitochondria [29].

Altogether, it is reasonable to conclude that the increased release of GSH into systemic circulation in CHD children who had undergone open heart surgery can be considered as a compensatory

Diagnostics **2019**, *9*, 118

mechanism to oxidative damage. The fact is of relevance bearing in mind that GSH is implicated the most in the protection against oxidative injury in glia, astrocytes, and neurons [30]. The mechanism through which GSH exerts its antioxidant action is, at this stage, not fully elucidated. One explanation resides in hypoxia or hyperoxia insults able to trigger the cellular GSH content, increasing the effect of N-acetylcysteine on repletion of GSH and further increasing key enzyme activities that regulate GSH production, glutamate cysteine ligase, and glutathione synthase [31,32]. In this light, it is reasonable to suggest that high GSH levels in blood may be the expression of a cascade of events affecting the glutathione/glutathione-oxidized ratio, which is hypoxia or hyperoxia mediated. Of note, high GSH levels in systemic circulation enhance its antioxidant capacity, thus reducing the proteins' defense mechanisms by oxidative damage. Another explanation resides in therapeutic strategies performed in the perioperative period such as transfusions (red blood cells, platelets), which contribute to redox imbalance being an important source of RNOS [33,34]. Finally, the possibility that therapeutic strategies such as anesthesia and fluid balance management can somewhat affect GSH levels must be taken into account. The fact is of relevance bearing in mind that (i) perioperative therapeutic strategies performed did not contain any thiol group, and (ii) fluid management was not responsible for any hemodilution/concentration phenomenon. Since no significant differences in Hb and Ht rate were observed at monitoring time points, these findings argue against the hypothesis.

In the present study, we also found that GSH increases in the perioperative period as PaO_2 peaks. Therefore, in order to limit the potential influence of oxygenation on GSH levels, we calculated the PaO_2/GSH ratio. The PaO_2/GSH ratio pattern increased during surgery up to the end of the procedure when it started to decrease, being superimposable to preoperative levels. The PaO_2/GSH ratio showed a positive correlation with CPB duration, cross-clamping, and body core temperature.

The finding of a correlation between GSH and PaO_2 deserves further consideration. In particular, increased GSH has shown the following: (i) in animal models, controlled normoxic reoxygenation limited brain injury [35]; (ii) in CHD children, lipid peroxidation increased and antioxidant reserve capacity decreased, being maintained by endogenous radical scavengers such as GSH [35–40]; and (iii) during CPB, increased oxygen toxicity affected endothelial permeability [2,35]. Altogether, it is reasonable to suggest that the higher GSH levels occurring during systemic reoxygenation in CHD children may be indicative of a compensatory mechanism due to CPB and hyperoxia-mediated stress.

Lastly, we found that the PaO_2/GSH ratio was superimposable to the one detected at the preoperative time point. The explanation may reside in the decay of PaO_2 levels at 24 h after surgery and explained by the short half-life of GSH (about 10 min) [41].

Finally, the present study shows some limitations. The main ones reside in the small population studied that did not allow to correct for the occurrence of cyanotic and non-cyanotic CHD and in the lack of an expanded oxidative stress evaluation with other biomarkers such as glutathione disulfide, non-protein bind iron and lipid hydroperoxides. Further studies in this regard are awaited.

In conclusion, the present data on elevated GSH levels, in CHD children undergoing open heart surgery and CPB, suggest that caution is needed in controlling different CPB phases such as DHCA, core body temperature, and systemic reoxygenation in a population that is per se more prone to CNS stress or damage. The findings may lead to further investigation to detect the "optimal" temperature and PaO_2 target [40] by monitoring biomarkers as much as possible to avoid perioperative CNS stress or damage.

Author Contributions: A.S. contributed to conceptualization, investigation, and writing—original draft. S.F. contributed to conceptualization, investigation, and writing—review and editing. G.L., F.P., L.A., E.B., and G.L. contributed to investigation and conceptualization. D.G. contributed to project administration, conceptualization, investigation, supervision, and writing—review and editing. All authors approved the final manuscript as submitted and agreed to be accountable for all aspects of the work.

Funding: This work is part of the I.O. PhD International Program under the auspices of the Italian Society of Neonatology and the Neonatal Clinical Biochemistry Research Group, and was partially supported by grants to D.G. from "I Colori della Vita Foundation", Italy.

Acknowledgments: The authors wish to thank Diasorin, Saluggia, Italy, for providing analysis kits.

Diagnostics **2019**, *9*, 118

Conflicts of Interest: The authors have no conflicts of interest relevant to this article to disclose.

Employment or Leadership: None declared.

Honorarium: The authors have no financial relationships relevant to this article to disclose.

Competing Interests: The funding organizations played no role in the study design; in the collection, analysis, and interpretation of data; in the writing of the report; or in the decision to submit the report for publication.

Abbreviation List

BE	base excess
BP	blood pressure
CHD	congenital heart disease
CPB	cardiopulmonary bypass
DHCA	deep hypothermic circulatory arrest
DTNB	2,2-dithio-bis-nitrobenzoic acid
GSH	glutathione
Hb	hemoglobin
HCO$_3$	bicarbonate
HR	heart rate
Ht	hematocrit rate
LA BP	left atrium BP
MUF	Modified ultrafiltration
PaCO$_2$	arterial carbon dioxide partial pressure
PaO$_2$	arterial oxygen partial pressure
RA BP	right atrium BP
RNOS	reactive nitrogen and oxygen species
SaO$_2$	pulsed arterial oxygenation
VSD	ventricular septal defect

References

1. Hsia, T.Y.; Gruber, P.J. Factors influencing neurologic out-come after neonatal cardiopulmonary bypass: What we can and cannot control. *Ann. Thorac. Surg.* **2006**, *81*, S2381–S2388. [CrossRef] [PubMed]
2. Gazzolo, D.; Abella, R.; Marinoni, E.; Di Iorio, R.; Livolti, G.; Galvano, F.; Pongiglione, G.; Frigiola, A.; Bertino, E.; Florio, P. Circulating biochemical markers of brain damage in infants complicated by ischemia reperfusion injury. *Cardiovasc. Hematol. Agents Med. Chem.* **2009**, *7*, 108–126. [CrossRef] [PubMed]
3. Guo, R.; Hou, W.; Dong, Y.; Yu, Z.; Stites, J.; Weiner, C.P. Brain injury caused by chronic fetal hypoxemia is mediated by inflammatory cascade activation. *Reprod. Sci.* **2010**, *17*, 540–548. [PubMed]
4. Adamy, C.; Mulder, P.; Khouzami, L.; Andrieu-Abadie, N.; Defer, N.; Candiani, G.; Pavoine, C.; Caramelle, P.; Souktani, R.; Le Corvoisier, P.; et al. Neutral sphingomyelinase inhibition participates to the benefits of Nacetylcysteine treatment in post-myocardial infarction failing heart rats. *J. Mol. Cell Cardiol.* **2007**, *43*, 344–353. [CrossRef] [PubMed]
5. Yucel, D.; Aydogdu, S.; Cehreli, S.; Saydam, G.; Canatan, H.; Senes, M.; Ciğdem Topkaya, B.; Nebioğlu, S. Increased oxidative stress in dilated cardiomyopathic heart failure. *Clin. Chem.* **1998**, *44*, 148–154.
6. Haddad, J.J.; Harb, H.L. L-gamma-Glutamyl-L-cysteinyl-glycine (glutathione; GSH) and GSH-related enzymes in the regulation of pro- and anti-inflammatory cytokines: A signaling transcriptional scenario for redox(y) immunologic sensor(s)? *Mol. Immunol.* **2005**, *42*, 987–1014. [CrossRef] [PubMed]
7. Franco, R.; Schoneveld, O.J.; Pappa, A.; Panayiotidis, M.I. The central role of glutathione in the pathophysiology of human diseases. *Arch. Physiol. Biochem.* **2007**, *113*, 234–258. [CrossRef] [PubMed]
8. Bourraindeloup, M.; Adamy, C.; Candiani, G.; Cailleret, M.; Bourin, M.C.; Badoual, T.; Su, J.B.; Adubeiro, S.; Roudot-Thoraval, F.; Dubois-Randé, J.L.; et al. N-acetylcysteine treatment normalizes serum tumor necrosis factor-alpha level and hinders the progression of cardiac injury in hypertensive rats. *Circulation* **2004**, *110*, 2003–2009. [CrossRef]

9. Damy, T.; Kirsch, M.; Khouzami, L.; Caramelle, P.; Le Corvoisier, P.; Roudot-Thoraval, F.; Dubois-Randé, J.L.; Hittinger, L.; Pavoine, C.; Pecker, F. Glutathione deficiency in cardiac patients is related to the functional status and structural cardiac abnormalities. *PLoS ONE* **2009**, *4*, e4871. [CrossRef]

10. Hayes, J.D.; McLellan, L.I. Glutathione and glutathione-dependent enzymes represent a co-ordinately regulated defence against oxidative stress. *Free Radic. Res.* **1999**, *31*, 273–300. [CrossRef]

11. Miyamoto, Y.; Koh, Y.H.; Park, Y.S.; Fujiwara, N.; Sakiyama, H.; Misonou, Y.; Ookawara, T.; Suzuki, K.; Honke, K.; Taniguchi, N. Oxidative stress caused by inactivation of glutathione peroxidase and adaptive responses. *Biol. Chem.* **2003**, *384*, 567–574. [CrossRef] [PubMed]

12. Huber, W.W.; Parzefall, W. Thiols and the chemoprevention of cancer. *Curr. Opin. Pharmacol.* **2007**, *7*, 404–409. [CrossRef] [PubMed]

13. Ciocoiu, M.; Badescu, M.; Paduraru, I. Protecting antioxidative effects of vitamins E and C in experimental physical stress. *J. Physiol. Biochem.* **2007**, *63*, 187–194. [CrossRef] [PubMed]

14. Hadzic, T.; Li, L.; Cheng, N.; Walsh, S.A.; Spitz, D.R.; Knudson, C.M. The role of low molecular weight thiols in T lymphocyte proliferation and IL-2 secretion. *J. Immunol.* **2005**, *175*, 7965–7972. [CrossRef] [PubMed]

15. Calza, G.; Lerzo, F.; Perfumo, F.; Borini, I.; Panizzon, G.; Moretti, R.; Grasso, P.; Virgone, A.; Zannini, L. Clinical evaluation of oxidative stress and myocardial reperfusion injury in pediatric cardiac surgery. *J. Cardiovasc. Surg. (Torino)* **2002**, *43*, 441–447.

16. Abella, R.; Satriano, A.; Frigiola, A.; Varrica, A.; Gavilanes, D.W.A.; Zimmermann, L.J.; Vles, H.J.S.; Florio, P.; Calevo, M.G.; Gazzolo, D. Adrenomedullin alterations related to cardiopulmonary bypass in infants with low cardiac output syndrome. *J. Matern. Fetal Neonatal Med.* **2012**, *25*, 2756–2761. [CrossRef] [PubMed]

17. Ziyaeifard, M.; Alizadehasl, A.; Massoumi, G. Modified ultrafiltration during cardiopulmonary bypass and postoperative course of pediatric cardiac surgery. *Res. Cardiovasc. Med.* **2014**, *3*, e17830.

18. Hu, M. Measurement of protein thiol groups and glutathione in plasma. *Methods Enzymol.* **1994**, *233*, 380–382.

19. Prechtl, H.F.R. Assessment methods for the newborn infant: A critical evaluation. In *Psychobiology of Human Newborn*; Stratton, D., Ed.; Wiley Chichester: London, UK, 1982; pp. 21–52.

20. Strobel, A.M.; Lu le, N. The Critically ill infant with congenital heart disease. *Emerg. Med. Clin. North. Am.* **2015**, *33*, 501–518. [CrossRef]

21. Kansy, A.; Tobota, Z.; Maruszewski, P.; Maruszewski, B. Analysis of 14,843 neonatal congenital heart surgical procedures in the European Association for Cardiothoracic Surgery congenital database. *Ann. Thorac. Surg.* **2010**, *89*, 1255–1259. [CrossRef]

22. Serpero, L.D.; Bellissima, V.; Colivicchi, M.; Sabatini, M.; Frigiola, A.; Ricotti, A.; Ghiglione, V.; Strozzi, M.C.; Livolti, G.; Galvano, F.; et al. Next generation biomarkers for brain injury. *J. Matern. Fetal Neonatal Med.* **2013**, *26*, 44–49. [CrossRef] [PubMed]

23. Abella, R.; Varrica, A.; Satriano, A.; Tettamanti, G.; Pelissero, G.; Gavilanes, A.D.; Zimmermann, L.J.; Vles, H.J.; Strozzi, M.C.; Pluchinotta, F.R.; et al. Biochemical markers for brain injury monitoring in children with or without congenital heart diseases. *Cns. Neurol. Disord. Drug Targets* **2015**, *14*, 12–23. [CrossRef] [PubMed]

24. Gazzolo, D.; Abella, R.; Marinoni, E.; Di Iorio, R.; Livolti, G.; Galvano, F.; Frigiola, A.; Temporini, F.; Moresco, L.; Colivicchi, M.; et al. New markers of neonatal neurology. *J. Matern Fetal Neonatal Med.* **2009**, *22*, 57–61. [CrossRef]

25. Gazzolo, D.; Michetti, F.; Bruschettini, M.; Marchese, N.; Lituania, M.; Mangraviti, S.; Pedrazzi, E.; Bruschettini, P. Pediatric concentrations of S100B protein in blood: age- and sex-related changes. *Clin. Chem.* **2003**, *49*, 967–970. [CrossRef] [PubMed]

26. McDonald, C.I.; Fraser, J.F.; Coombes, J.S.; Fung, Y.L. Oxidative stress during extracorporeal circulation. *Eur J. Cardiothorac Surg.* **2014**, *46*, 937–943. [CrossRef] [PubMed]

27. Türker, F.S.; Doğan, A.; Ozan, G.; Kıbar, K.; Erışır, M. Change in free radical and antioxidant enzyme levels in the patients undergoing open heart surgery with cardiopulmonary bypass. *Oxid. Med. Cell Longev.* **2016**, *2016*, 1783728. [CrossRef] [PubMed]

28. Alva, N.; Azuara, D.; Palomeque, J.; Carbonell, T. Deep hypothermia protects against acute hypoxia in vivo in rats: A mechanism related to the attenuation of oxidative stress. *Exp. Physiol.* **2013**, *98*, 1115–1124. [CrossRef]

29. Turrens, J.F.; Freeman, B.A.; Crapo, J.D. Hyperoxia increases H_2O_2 release by lung mitochondria and microsomes. *Arch. Biochem. Biophys.* **1982**, *217*, 411–421. [CrossRef]

30. Ben-Yoseph, O.; Boxer, P.A.; Ross, B.D. Assessment of the role of the glutathione and pentose phosphate pathways in the protection of primary cerebrocortical cultures from oxidative stress. *J. Neurochem.* **1996**, *66*, 2329–2337. [CrossRef]

31. Rahman, Q.; Abidi, P.; Afaq, F.; Schiffmann, D.; Mossman, B.T.; Kamp, D.W.; Athar, M. Glutathione redox system in oxidative lung injury. *Crit. Rev. Toxicol.* **1999**, *29*, 543–568. [CrossRef]

32. Ko, Y.E.; Lee, I.H.; So, H.M.; Kim, H.V.; Kim, Y.H. Mechanism of glutathione depletion during simulated ischemia-reperfusion of H9c2 cardiac myocytes. *Free Radic. Res.* **2011**, *45*, 1074–1082. [CrossRef]

33. Rosa, S.; Bristor, M.; Topanotti, M.; Tomasi, C.; Felisberto, F.; Vuolo, F.; Petronilho, F.; Pizzol, F.D.; Ritter, C. Effect of red cell transfusion on parameters of inflammation and oxidative stress in critically ill patients. *Rev. Bras. Ter. Intensiva.* **2011**, *23*, 30–35. [CrossRef]

34. Krotz, F.; Sohn, H.Y.; Pohl, U. Reactive oxygen species: Players in the platelet game. *Arter. Thromb Vasc Biol.* **2004**, *24*, 1988–1996. [CrossRef]

35. Buckberg, G.D. Studies of hypoxemic/reoxygenation injury: I. Linkage between cardiac function and oxidant damage. *J. Thorac. Cardiovasc. Surg.* **1995**, *110*, 1164–1170. [CrossRef]

36. Kirklin, J.W.; Barratt-Boyes, B.G. *Cardiac surgery: Morphology, Diagnostic Criteria, Natural History, Techniques, Results and Indication*; Churchill Livingston Inc.: New York, NY, USA, 1993; p. 77.

37. Morita, K.; Ihnken, K.; Buckberg, G.D. Studies of hypoxemic/reoxygenation injury: With aortic clamping. XII. Delay of cardiac reoxygenation damage in the presence of cyanosis: A new concept of controlled cardiac reoxygenation. *J. Thorac. Cardiovasc. Surg.* **1995**, *110*, 1265–1273. [CrossRef]

38. Del Nido, P.J.; Mickle, D.A.; Wilson, G.J.; Benson, M.L.; Coles, J.G.; Trusler, G.A.; Williams, W.G. Evidence of myocardial free radical injury during elective repair of tetralogy of Fallot. *Circulation* **1987**, *76*, V174–V179.

39. Schurr, A. Lactate, glucose and energy metabolism in the ischemic brain. *Int J. Mol Med.* **2002**, *10*, 131–136. [CrossRef]

40. Arrica, M.; Bissonnette, B. Therapeutic hypothermia. *Semin. Cardiothorac. Vasc. Anesth.* **2007**, *11*, 6–15. [CrossRef]

41. Hong, S.Y.; Gil, H.W.; Yang, J.O.; Lee, E.Y.; Kim, H.K.; Kim, S.H.; Chung, Y.H.; Hwang, S.K.; Lee, Z.W. Pharmacokinetics of glutathione and its metabolites in normal subjects. *J. Korean Med. Sci.* **2005**, *20*, 721–726. [CrossRef]

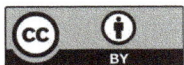

diagnostics

MDPI

Article

An Easy and Reliable Strategy for Making Type I Interferon Signature Analysis Comparable among Research Centers

Alessia Pin [1], Lorenzo Monasta [2], Andrea Taddio [1,3], Elisa Piscianz [4], Alberto Tommasini [3,* and Alessandra Tesser [4]

[1] Department of Medicine, Surgery and Health Sciences, University of Trieste, 34127 Trieste, Italy
[2] Clinical Epidemiology and Public Health Research Unit, Institute for Maternal and Child Health—IRCCS "Burlo Garofolo", 34137 Trieste, Italy
[3] Department of Paediatrics, Institute for Maternal and Child Health—IRCCS "Burlo Garofolo", 34137 Trieste, Italy
[4] Department of Advanced Diagnostic and Clinical Trials, Institute for Maternal and Child Health—IRCCS "Burlo Garofolo", 34137 Trieste, Italy
* Correspondence: alberto.tommasini@burlo.trieste.it

Received: 9 August 2019; Accepted: 3 September 2019; Published: 4 September 2019

Abstract: Interferon-stimulated genes (ISGs) are a set of genes whose transcription is induced by interferon (IFN). The measure of the expression of ISGs enables calculating an IFN score, which gives an indirect estimate of the exposition of cells to IFN-mediated inflammation. The measure of the IFN score is proposed for the screening of monogenic interferonopathies, like the Aicardi-Goutières syndrome, or to stratify subjects with systemic lupus erythematosus to receive IFN-targeted treatments. Apart from these scenarios, there is no agreement on the diagnostic value of the score in distinguishing IFN-related disorders from diseases dominated by other types of cytokines. Since the IFN score is currently measured in several research hospitals, merging experiences could help define the potential of scoring IFN inflammation in clinical practice. However, the IFN score calculated at different laboratories may be hardly comparable due to the distinct sets of IFN-stimulated genes assessed and to different controls used for data normalization. We developed a reliable approach to minimize the inter-laboratory variability, thereby providing shared strategies for the IFN signature analysis and allowing different centers to compare data and merge their experiences.

Keywords: interferon signature score; inter-laboratory variability; data sharing; systemic lupus erythematosus; interferonopathies; biostatistics

1. Introduction

Type I interferon (IFN) production is part of the innate immune response to viruses or intracellular bacteria, which is triggered by the sensing of pathogen-associated nucleic acids [1]. Even though the identification of IFNs dates back to the 50s–60s [2], the description of a group of mendelian disorders with dysregulated IFN-mediated inflammation has only recently shed light on the fine regulation of the production and action of these cytokines [3]. Of note, this new group of disorders, known as type I interferonopathies, displays significant phenotypic overlaps with both systemic lupus erythematosus (SLE) and congenital viral infections of the TORCH (Toxoplasmosis, Rubella, Cytomegalovirus, Herpes simplex) and HIV (human immunodeficiency virus) groups [3,4].

Type I interferonopathies are marked by the hyper-expression of a set of genes (IFN-stimulated genes, ISGs) in inflamed tissue and often in peripheral blood, leading to the definition of the so-called "IFN signature" [5,6]. The IFN signature was firstly defined in subjects with SLE to assess the level of IFN related inflammation and to help stratify patients to receive IFN targeted treatments [7–9].

Since then, the measure of expression of the ISGs (IFN signature analysis) is increasingly used in biomedical research centers, as well as for the functional classification of other conditions characterized by a type I IFN dysregulation [10], to distinguish such conditions from classical inflammatory disorders predominantly mediated by other cytokines, like Tumor Necrosis Factor α and Interleukin 1 (i.e., inflammatory bowel diseases, rheumatoid arthritis, and periodic fevers) [11].

Different ISG sets were identified to evaluate interferon-mediated autoinflammation and are frequently restricted to 5-6 targeted genes [6,10,12,13], suitable, for example, for the discrimination of Aicardi-Goutières syndrome (AGS) [6,10]. However, IFN signature analysis could be extended to larger gene lists [7] or even restricted to just one single gene, particularly when directly assessed in affected tissues, as in the case of dermatomyositis [14–16].

Even though the IFN signature measure has become widely available at research hospitals, there is no consensus for the selection of calibration controls. Thus, it is hard to compare data among distinct centers and to estimate the potential of IFN signature testing for discriminating among inflammatory conditions in the clinical practice. For example, thousands of subjects with antiphospholipid syndrome have been described in multicenter studies [17], while the interferon score has been separately studied in several small series without allowing the merging of results [18–22].

The main problem hindering the use of IFN signature analysis for in vitro diagnostics is the expression of data relativized to independent healthy control(s) in each laboratory, leading to unpredictable inter-laboratory variability. It is logical to assume that the use of pooled cDNA from healthy donors can represent a convenient strategy for calibrating Real Time quantitative PCR (qPCR) for the assessment of the IFN score. However, it can be difficult to predict the optimal number of samples to be pooled, which requires minimizing variability between one pool and another prepared at distinct laboratories, as already pointed out by others [23,24].

This study aims to investigate, through laboratory, bioinformatic, and statistical analyses, a reliable approach to minimize the variability that can be observed in inter-laboratory assays.

The final goal is providing shared recommendations for IFN signature analysis and interpretation of data in the clinical practice, thereby allowing data sharing among reference centers and improving knowledge on IFN-related disorders.

2. Materials and Methods

The study is part of the IRCCS Burlo Garofolo project RC #24/2017, approved by the Institutional Review Board and by the Friuli Venezia Giulia Independent Ethical Committee (2018-SPER-079-BURLO, N. 0039851, approved on 12 December 2018). All investigations were performed after obtaining written informed consent from volunteers and patients or their parents/guardians.

2.1. Subjects

On wet IFN signature analysis was assessed by quantitative PCR (qPCR) in ten young-aged healthy subjects (Dataset A, ten out of eleven individuals, five males and five females).

To establish whether data from qPCR and RNAseq analysis were comparable, IFN signature on wet (by qPCR) and in silico (by RNAseq) analysis was performed in twenty subjects with inflammatory diseases, such as systemic lupus erythematosus (SLE), interferonopathies or inflammatory bowel diseases (IBD), and patients' relatives, recruited at our center (Dataset E). A brief description of patients' clinical diagnosis is displayed in Table S1.

To increase healthy donors numerosity, in silico IFN signature investigation (by RNAseq) has been performed in twenty healthy individuals, collected at our center Dataset A (four out of eleven individuals), and selected from different whole blood RNA-sequencing (RNAseq) open-access web-based datasets: we sorted another three datasets, while considering exclusively healthy control samples, accessible at ArrayExpress (accession number E-MTAB-5735, Dataset B, five individuals) and at the Gene Expression Omnibus (GEO) (accession number GSE112057, Dataset C, nine individuals; GSE90081, Dataset D, two individuals). Specification about gender was not available for all the samples. However, sex has been easily inferred by expression analysis of the sex-specific genes *RPS4Y1* and *USP9Y*.

The dataset composition is shown in Table 1.

Table 1. Dataset composition: subjects, size, methods and purposes.

Datasets	Subjects	*n* Total (F/M)	Method (*n*)	Purpose
A—Data of from our center; Accession: #	Healthy donors	11 (5/6)	qPCR (10) RNAseq (3)	To test the variability of expression of the six ISGs in a healthy donor small group available at out center
			RNAseq (1)	To increase the healthy donor group size, to improve the power of the variability measurement
B—Accession: E-MTAB-5735	Healthy donors	5 (2/3)	RNAseq (5)	To increase the healthy donor group size, to improve the power of the variability measurement
C—Accession: GSE112057	Healthy donors	12 (6/6)	RNAseq (9)	To increase the healthy donor group size, to improve the power of the variability measurement
D—Accession: GSE90081	Healthy donors	12 (12/0)	RNAseq (2)	To increase the healthy donor group size, to improve the power of the variability measurement
E—Patients and patient's relatives recruited at our center	Patients	20 (9/11)	qPCR (20) RNAseq (20)	To compare IFN signature results between qPCR and RNAseq analyses

data not present in open-access web-based datasets.

2.2. Sample Collection, RNA Isolation and cDNA Preparation

Peripheral blood was collected in PAXgene Blood RNA Tubes (PreAnalytiX, Hombrechtikon, Switzerland) and, after two-hours incubation at room temperature, tubes were frozen at −20 °C until processing. Total RNA was extracted with PAXgene Blood RNA Kit (PreAnalytiX, Switzerland), following the manufacturer's instructions, and quantified with NanoDrop Spectrophotometer (Thermo Fisher, Waltham, MA, USA). RNA integrity was checked using an Agilent Technologies 2100 Bioanalyzer.

Up to 1 μg of total RNA was retro-transcribed using SensiFAST cDNA Synthesis Kit (Bioline, London, UK).

2.3. IFN Signature Analysis

The expression of six IFN-stimulated genes was assessed by qPCR using AB 7500 Real Time PCR System (Applied Biosystems, Waltham, MA, USA), TaqMan Gene Expression Master Mix (Applied Biosystems, USA) and UPL Probes (Roche, Basel, Switzerland) for *IFI27, IFI44L, IFIT1, ISG15, RSAD2*, and *SIGLEC1*. Using AB 7500 Real Time PCR software, each target quantity was normalized with the expression level of *HPRT1* and *G6PD*, and the relative quantification (RQ) was conducted relating to a "calibrator" sample (mix of ten healthy controls, Dataset A) using the $2^{-\Delta\Delta Ct}$ method [25]. The median fold change of the six genes was used to calculate the IFN score for each patient.

2.4. RNAseq Analysis

Transcriptome sequencing was performed using the TruSeq Stranded mRNA Sample Preparation kit (Illumina, San Diego, CA, USA) and sequenced on a NovaSeq 6000 platform (Illumina, San Diego, CA, USA), generating 2X100 bp paired-end reads (30 million reads per sample) in twenty subjects from Dataset E (patients and patients' relatives) and four out of eleven controls from Dataset A.

RNAseq raw data (either our data and open-access web-based data) workflow was conducted as follows: quality control by FastQC (https://www.bioinformatics.babraham.ac.uk/projects/fastqc/), quality filtering by Trim Galore (https://www.bioinformatics.babraham.ac.uk/projects/trim_galore/), read alignment to hg38 using annotation from GENECODE v.31 (https://www.gencodegenes.org/) with STAR [26], reads counting into genes by featureCounts [27].

Data of patients with autoinflammatory diseases and three healthy individuals of our dataset were normalized and analyzed for differentially expressed genes by DESeq2 [28]. From the result table, we only considered the ISGs and evaluated their relative fold changes on each patient compared to the set of controls.

To assess the ISGs expression variability within the group of twenty healthy subjects, shortlisted from the datasets described above, we determined the expression values for each gene, normalized by Fragments Per Kilobase per Million mapped reads (FPKM) method with edgeR (*rpkm* function) [29,30], using the values from the "Length" column, in the featureCounts' output, for the calculation.

Principal component analysis (PCA), useful for data visualization, was conducted with DESeq2, to define the overall variability between samples.

2.5. Statistical Analyses

Considering that each of the six genes measured was expressed on a different scale, we decided to calculate the sample size based on the coefficient of variation, instead than the mean and the standard deviation. We further hypothesized that different runs did not increase the variation in comparing the samples, assuming the only origin of variability to be represented by the subjects' heterogeneity.

To determine the statistical power for data obtained by qPCR and RNAseq, we computed the noncentrality parameter (λ) using GPower 3.1.9.2. software [31,32], with a generic two-tailed *t*-test, given $\alpha = 0.05$, $\beta = 0.2$, and degrees of freedom equal N-1. If the noncentrality parameter under these conditions (reference value, "λref") resulted in being lower than the one calculated on our samples, we considered the sample size as appropriate.

GraphPad Prism 6 software was employed for χ^2 contingency analysis; *p*-values <0.05 were considered significant.

To identify the appropriate sample size for variability assessment, we computed λ for increasing numerosity (up to forty) using GPower 3.1.9.2. (Heinrich-Heine University Düsseldorf, Germany), and determined a "plateau value" by an exponential decay function (GraphPad Prism 6 software, La Jolla California USA).

3. Results

3.1. Variability Assessment in IFN-Stimulated Genes Expression in Healthy Controls (Dataset A) Analyzed by qPCR

The variability of expression of the six ISGs (*IFI27*, *IFI44L*, *IFIT1*, *ISG15*, *RSAD2*, *SIGLEC1*) was assessed in ten healthy controls processed by on wet qPCR analysis. Five out of six genes showed low variability coefficients and noncentrality parameters (λ) that fulfilled the analysis criteria (as described in Materials and Methods, Section 2.5) (Table 2). Only *IFI44L* did not comply with the analysis parameters, presenting higher variability and a lower λ than the reference value (λref) (Figure 1)

Table 2. Variability assessment for interferon-stimulated genes (ISGs) expression values quantified in ten out of eleven healthy subjects from Dataset A by qPCR.

	IFI27	IFI44L	IFIT1	ISG15	RSAD2	SIGLEC1
Mean	4.57	0.72	2.18	4.61	1.24	5.14
SD	1.04	0.91	1.05	0.60	1.20	0.42
Variability coefficient	0.23	1.26	0.48	0.13	0.96	0.08
λ ($n = 10$)	13.92	**2.52**	6.56	24.47	3.28	38.99
λref: 3.15						

SD: standard deviation; λref: noncentrality parameter (λ) calculated based on $\alpha = 0.05$, $\beta = 0.2$, and degrees of freedom equal N-1. Sample size is considered as appropriate when λ computed on each gene is higher than λref. The value below λref is highlighted in bold.

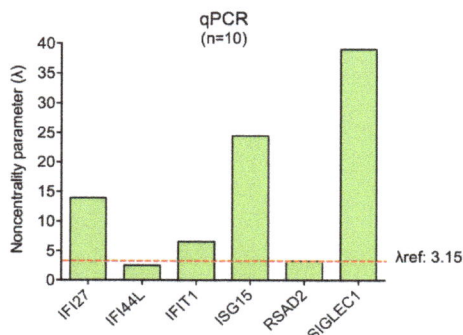

Figure 1. Graphical representation of the noncentrality parameter (λ) calculated for each ISG by on wet qPCR analysis. The λref for ten subjects is displayed by the dashed line and reported in the figure. Sample size is considered as appropriate when λ computed on each gene is higher than λref.

Thus, ten healthy controls could not be considered an appropriate sample size to represent an ideal healthy population, in which the physiologically floating expression values of the ISGs present acceptable variability. For this reason, we should increase the numerosity of healthy controls to obtain a suitable pool in which the gene expression variability is minimized.

3.2. IFN-Stimulated Genes Expression Evaluated by qPCR or RNAseq Analysis Are Comparable

To improve the power of the variability measurement, we decided to take advantage of RNAseq open-access web-based data, as an easy source to increase the number of healthy subjects to calculate ISGs interindividual differences. This choice came from comparisons between the relative ISGs fold change assessed in the same twenty subjects (Dataset E) by both qPCR and RNAseq analysis, selecting the same set of three out of eleven healthy controls from Dataset A, to normalize data for both techniques.

Some subjects showed different relative expression values for the same gene calculated by on wet qPCR and in silico RNAseq, but the overall results of the IFN signatures (IFN scores) were extremely consistent between the two techniques for each individual (χ^2 contingency analysis *p*-value = 0.405, not significant). The comparability of IFN scores is easily explained, considering that these values represent the median of the six relative ISGs quantifications, and they broadly reflect the overexpression status in the analyzed sample (Table 3). Thus, the two methods provided the same trend in gene expression in subjects presenting low, intermediate, and high IFN signatures, as indicated by the three representative graphs in Figure 2 (Subject n.9: low IFN signature; Subject n.14: intermediate IFN signature; Subject n.11: high IFN signature).

Table 3. Comparison of interferon (IFN) scores determined in twenty subjects by both qPCR and RNAseq by χ^2 contingency analysis (*p*-value = 0.405, not significant).

Subject *n.*	IFN Score	
	In Silico RNAseq	On Wet qPCR
1	3.26	5.01
2	6.79	10.05
3	7.12	9.85
4	8.58	10.74
5	1.55	1.37
6	1.11	0.97
7	0.55	0.67
8	0.22	0.19
9	1.14	1.05
10	3.68	2.60
11	77.73	82.61
12	44.03	94.25
13	17.44	16.48
14	15.44	16.35
15	37.43	49.98
16	37.44	84.99
17	1.07	1.18
18	2.39	4.70
19	3.01	1.71
20	1.82	1.82
Mean	19.83	13.59
SD	31.19	20.33
Variability coefficient	1.57	1.50

SD: standard deviation.

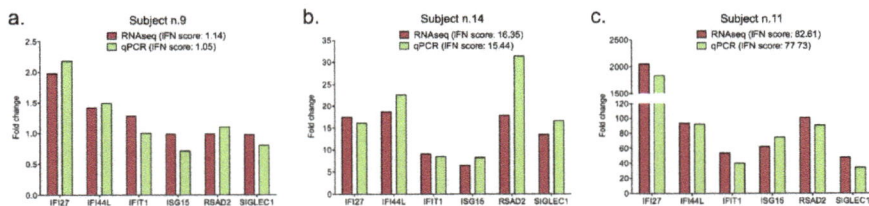

Figure 2. Representative display of low (**a**), intermediate (**b**) and high (**c**) IFN signatures analyzed by both qPCR and RNAseq for each subject. For the optimal graphical representation of all histograms, the scales of values are set different. The IFN scores computed for each subject are reported in the legend of the figures.

3.3. Preliminary Analysis for Sample Selection and Variability Assessment in IFN-Stimulated Genes Expression Analyzed by RNAseq

Given the comparability of data between qPCR and RNAseq, we exploited the availability of large open-access web repositories containing RNAseq data to calculate the proper sample size for the assessment of the IFN score with an acceptable inter-laboratory variability.

To select the appropriate sample size, we firstly calculated the noncentrality parameter (λ) on a numerosity up to forty individuals using GPower software. Then, we determine the plateau value of the exponential decay function of the previously computed λ values. The provided plateau (3.01) corresponds to λ for sample size $n = 15$ (Figure 3), leading us to consider fifteen subjects as an appropriate sample size. For more experimental strength, we considered both $n = 15$ and $n = 20$ in the following analyses. We did not further increase the sample size over twenty subjects, whereas exceeding this number might bring difficulties in term of donors' collection.

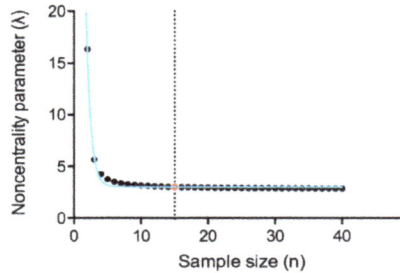

Figure 3. Plateau value (reported as a red dot) threshold (reported as a dotted vertical line) of λ computed for sample sizes up to forty subjects. Each sample size is represented by a black dot. In blue the exponential decay function curve of the previously computed λ.

We performed a principal component analysis (PCA), a data visualization analysis, to evaluate the total expression variation of the six ISGs and to define the most homogeneous set of twenty healthy individuals. This investigation allows the detection of possible rare outliers with the highest variance that might not be considered as suitable controls to study IFN signature.

RNAseq records have been chosen considering the presence of similar features such as blood collection type, RNA extraction protocol and library selection, to reduce as much as possible the technical procedure variability (Table 3).

As a first attempt, we investigated all the RNAseq samples of healthy donors from Dataset A (data from our center, $n = 4/11$), Dataset B (E-MTAB-5735, $n = 5$) and Dataset C (GSE112057, $n = 12$), twenty-one specimens in total. Figure 4a displays the PCA results showing the overall ISGs expression variability between individuals. The analysis exhibited a higher variance in three out of twenty-one subjects: we thus decided not to include these three samples in further studies, collecting eighteen samples that were suitable for our purpose. To get the proper numerosity ($n = 20$), we examine Dataset D (GSE90081, $n = 12$) and we ran the same analysis again, obtaining a satisfactory level of variation, without outliers, between datasets and among individuals. From these preliminary observations, we randomly chose two out of twelve samples from Dataset D, combining them with data previously selected. Again, we observed an acceptable gene expression variability among our final twenty-controls-sized group (Table 4), as shown in Figure 4b.

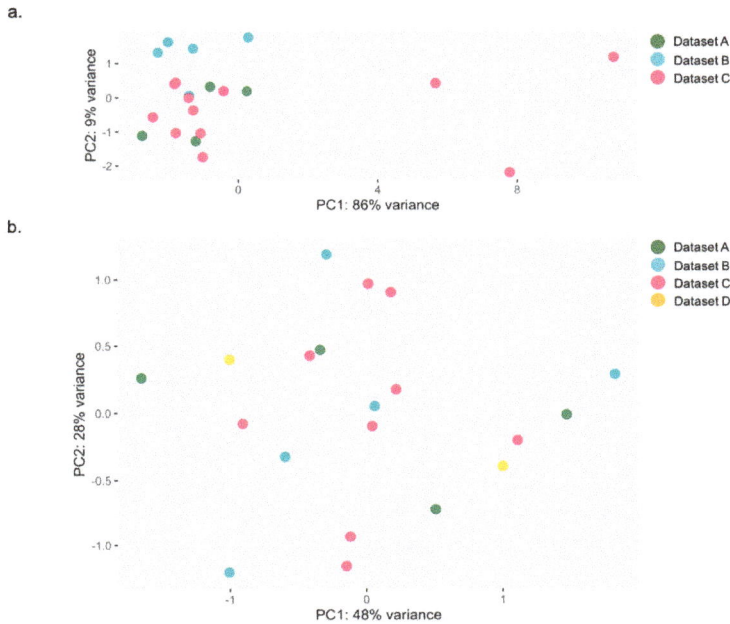

Figure 4. Overall ISGs expression variance between individuals. PCA of the first selection (**a**), with evidence of the three outliers from Dataset C, and of the final twenty-controls-sized group (**b**), showing twenty samples uniformly distributed (4 from Dataset A, 5 from Dataset B, 9 from Dataset C and 2 from Dataset D).

Table 4. Detailed report of final twenty-controls-sized healthy subject groups.

Datasets	Subjects				RNAseq Details	
Authors & Accession	Female ($n = 9$)	Male ($n = 11$)	Whole Blood collection/RNA extraction		RNAseq library preparation/platform	Read Length
A—Data from our center; Accession:#	2	2	PAXgene blood RNA tube/PAXgene Blood RNA Kit		Illumina TruSeq stranded mRNA library protocol/Novaseq	Paired-end 100 bp reads
B—Rodero MP, et al., 2017; Accession: E-MTAB-5735	2	3	PAXgene blood RNA tube/PAXgene Blood RNA Kit		Illumina TruSeq stranded mRNA library protocol/Illumina HiSeq 2000	Paired-end 75 bp reads
C—Mo A., et al., 2018; Accession: GSE112057	3	6	Tempus Tube/Tempus Spin isolation RNA kit		Illumina TruSeq stranded mRNA library protocol/Illumina HiSeq Rapid Run	Paired-end 100 bp reads
D—Shchetynsky K., et al., 2017; Accession: GSE90081	2	-	PAXgene blood RNA tube/PAXgene Blood miRNA kit		Standard illumina TruSeq RNA protocol, following PolyA enrichment/Illumina HiSeq 2000	Paired-end 100 bp reads

data not present in open-access web-based datasets.

We calculated the λref for larger samples of healthy controls (fifteen and twenty subjects) using GPower software, and the variability of the ISGs expression in fifteen and twenty healthy controls processed by in silico RNAseq analysis. Table 5 shows that all the variability coefficients are considerably low and all λ calculated fulfilled the analysis parameters (Figure 5) (expression values of single gene for each control are displayed in Table S2. Thus, we can hypothesize that pooling together samples from fifteen or twenty healthy subjects could also be considered a proper sample size in qPCR analyses.

Table 5. Variability assessment for IFN-stimulated genes expression values evaluated in fifteen and twenty healthy subjects by in silico RNAseq analysis.

		IFI27	IFI44L	IFIT1	ISG15	RSAD2	SIGLEC1
	Mean	0.35	1.14	5.06	30.17	2.21	1.17
	SD	0.23	0.28	1.29	12.44	0.86	0.55
$n = 15$	Variability coefficient	0.64	0.25	0.26	0.41	0.39	0.47
	λ	6.09	15.64	15.16	9.39	9.93	8.21
	Λref: 3.01						
	Mean	0.33	1.26	5.17	30.09	2.47	1.22
	SD	0.22	0.38	1.38	14.41	1.00	0.50
$n = 20$	Variability coefficient	0.67	0.30	0.27	0.48	0.41	0.41
	λ	6.68	14.70	16.77	9.34	10.98	10.90
	λref: 2.95						

SD: standard deviation; λref: noncentrality parameter calculated based on $\alpha = 0.05$, $\beta = 0.2$, and degrees of freedom equal N-1. Sample size is considered as appropriate when λ computed on each gene is higher than λref.

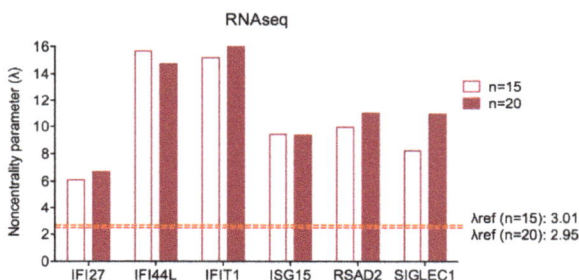

Figure 5. Graphical representation of λ calculated for each ISG by in silico RNAseq analysis. The λrefs for fifteen and twenty subjects are displayed by the red dashed line and reported in the figure. Sample size is considered appropriate when λ computed on each gene is higher than λref.

3.4. Pooling Twenty Subjects Could Be Considered an Optimal Strategy to Minimize Gene Expression Variability among Healthy Controls for on Wet IFN Signature Analysis

We checked whether the values of mean, SD and variability coefficient obtained by on wet qPCR on ten controls met the λ criteria considering $n = 15$ and $n = 20$ subjects as already calculated, assuming that the variability coefficient does not change as the sample size increases (Table 6).

Table 6. Estimated variability assessment for ISGs expression values in fifteen and twenty healthy subjects for qPCR analysis assuming the same variability coefficient for increasing sample size.

	IFI27	IFI44L	IFIT1	ISG15	RSAD2	SIGLEC1
Mean	4.57	0.72	2.18	4.61	1.24	5.14
SD	1.04	0.91	1.05	0.60	1.20	0.42
Variability coefficient	0.23	1.26	0.48	0.13	0.96	0.08
λ ($n = 15$)	17.05	3.08	8.04	29.97	4.02	47.75
λref: 3.01						
λ ($n = 20$)	19.69	3.56	9.28	34.61	4.64	55.14
λref: 2.95						

Mean, standard deviation (SD) and variability coefficient values previously determined on ten subjects are reported in the table. λref: noncentrality parameter (λ) calculated based on $\alpha = 0.05$, $\beta = 0.2$, and degrees of freedom equal N-1. Sample size is considered appropriate when λ computed on each gene is higher than λref.

The analysis provides quite good results for both sample sizes tested, even if *IFI44L* showed a λ (3.08) very close to λref (3.01). For this reason, we can consider more adequate to increase the numerosity to twenty subjects, a still easy-to-gather number of healthy donors. Thus, we could assert that twenty healthy controls could be considered a suitable sample size for IFN signature analysis performed by qPCR, as predicted by in silico RNAseq (Figure 6).

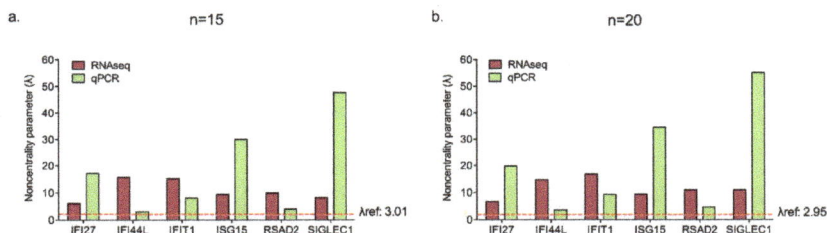

Figure 6. Graphical representation of λ calculated for each ISG by in silico RNAseq analysis and hypothesized qPCR assessment considering fifteen (**a**) and twenty (**b**) subjects. The λrefs values are displayed by the red dashed line and reported in the figure. Sample size is considered appropriate when λ computed on each gene is higher than λref.

4. Discussion

The clinical employment of the IFN signature is strictly related to the screening of pathological conditions characterized by type I IFN dysregulation [24]. However, several studies have been carried out to associate the IFN-related inflammation with specific clinical or laboratory features of rheumatologic conditions, like systemic lupus erythematosus, primary antiphospholipid syndrome, Sjögren syndrome, rheumatoid arthritis, autoimmune myositis and systemic sclerosis [18,20,33–38]. Some Authors proposed that the assessment of IFN inflammation may help identify subgroups of patients with a better response to specific treatments, as B cell targeted therapies [39–42]. Moreover, since most anti-inflammatory or immunomodulatory agents have only a weak effect on IFN inflammation, the calculation of the IFN score may also serve to guide targeted therapy approaches with novel drugs like Janus Kinase inhibitors [10].

However, there is no consensus on a shared and validated method to classify different inflammatory conditions by transcriptome analysis. Crow and collaborators used pooled cDNA from healthy donors as calibrator for qPCR, and after assessing a large number of healthy controls and patients with Aicardi-Goutières Syndrome calculated a fixed cut-off value of normality suitable for the screening of interferonopathies [6]. However, this cut-off has been validated to facilitate the detection of monogenic interferonopathies and not to assess IFN inflammation in other conditions. Moreover, the reference to locally pooled control cDNA may make it difficult to compare results obtained in distinct centers.

Even though multiple ISG panels have been described either in peripheral blood cells or affected tissues, many laboratories set their assays by analyzing a minimal set of 5-6 targeted-genes, usually including the set proposed by Crow et al. This set has been applied to thousands of analyses and its potential for screening of monogenic interferonopathies is established. After the normalization of results on at least two housekeeping genes, the main source of variability limiting interlaboratory comparison of data consists in the use of different controls for data normalization. Indeed, this is a remarkable problem, considering that the potential role of IFN signature analysis in clinical practice can be defined only by sharing data among research centers, comparing or merging case series. Of course, the best option for the future should rely on the development of industrially manufactured kits validated for In Vitro Diagnostics (IVD) and usable worldwide with the same reference values, not only in the most advanced research areas. Conversely, only the analysis and comparison of data available at various centers can tell industries whether the development of such diagnostic kits is worthwhile or not. Thus, we focused on a strategy that could be immediately applied in biomedical laboratories to facilitate the sharing of experience and minimize the inter-laboratory variability.

We investigated if using a pool of biological samples from healthy controls could solve the data normalization issue, which is the main source of inter-laboratory variability. We proposed that this strategy could "equalize" the differences in gene expression that physiologically occur among individuals.

For this purpose, we evaluated if any pool of healthy controls more than a given number n of subjects could be suitable to level differences, through an approach based on laboratory (qPCR), bioinformatic (RNAseq), and statistical data integration analyses.

Starting from the ISGs expression assessment in peripheral blood from ten healthy subjects by on wet qPCR analysis, we found that this sample size is not suitable for equalizing the variable expression levels of all the six ISGs in healthy volunteers. To find the appropriate number of samples to be pooled together with low enough variability, we further investigated if public data from RNAseq can be exploited to expand our analysis. We thus compared relative ISGs fold change values calculated by qPCR and RNAseq analysis for the same subjects with the same calibrator, showing that the two methods yield comparable results with very low variability between each other. Previous studies compared gene expression measurements generated by in silico RNAseq and on wet qPCR assays, showing consistent results between the two methods for most genes, with the only exception of some genes generally characterized by small size and low expression levels. None of the ISGs is included in the list of genes with inconsistent estimation of expression according to the Authors [43]. Our results confirmed that RNAseq and qPCR generate consistent results in the assessment of ISGs expression levels. Thus, based on the literature and on our preliminary results, we considered RNAseq as a good asset to increase the number of healthy subjects on which to calculate interindividual differences in ISGs expression, exploiting both RNAseq samples available at our center and open-access web-based data.

The results of our study support the choice of pooling twenty healthy controls for the normalization of the assay, allowing to express results as relative to a "standard set of controls". Of note, we validated this sample size only for the selected set of six ISGs in peripheral blood cells. The expression of other genes included in larger panels, may present higher variability among donors and between different affected tissues. However, the same procedure that we have described can also be used to define the optimal sample size for other transcription profiles, for interferonopathies or for other rheumatologic disorders. The performance of the proposed twenty-controls-sized standard could be improved by analyzing all the donors separately before pooling, and by performing cluster variance analysis, which can enable excluding rare donors with outlier variance.

Supplementary Materials: The following are available online at http://www.mdpi.com/2075-4418/9/3/113/s1.

Author Contributions: Conceptualization: A.T. (Alberto Tommasini), A.P. (Alessia Pin), A.T. (Alessandra Tesser); methodology: A.P. (Alessia Pin), A.T. (Alessandra Tesser), L.M.; software: A.P. (Alessia Pin), L.M.; validation: A.P. (Alessia Pin), A.T. (Alessandra Tesser), E.P.; resources: A.T. (Alberto Tommasini); data curation: A.P. (Alessia Pin), A.T. (Alessandra Tesser), L.M., E.P.; writing—original draft preparation: A.P. (Alessia Pin), A.T. (Alessandra Tesser), L.M.; writing—review and editing: A.T. (Alberto Tommasini), E.P., A.T. (Andrea Taddio); supervision: A.T. (Alberto Tommasini), A.T. (Andrea Taddio), E.P.; project administration: A.T. (Alberto Tommasini), A.T. (Andrea Taddio), A.T. (Alessandra Tesser); funding acquisition: A.T. (Alberto Tommasini), A.T. (Andrea Taddio).

Funding: This research was funded by the Institute for Maternal and Child Health IRCCS "Burlo Garofolo" RC #24/2017.

Acknowledgments: We thank Stefano Volpi from IRCCS Istituto Giannina Gaslini (Genova, Italy) for the long-term support and scientific confrontation and Remo Sanges from International School for Advanced Studies (SISSA, Trieste, Italy) for the bioinformatic analysis support.

Conflicts of Interest: The authors declare no conflict of interest.

References

1. Stetson, D.B.; Medzhitov, R. Type I interferons in host defense. *Immunity* **2006**, *25*, 373–381. [CrossRef] [PubMed]

2. Isaacs, A.; Lindenmann, J. Virus interference. I. The interferon. *Proc. R. Soc. Lond. B Biol. Sci.* **1957**, *147*, 258–267. [PubMed]

3. Crow, Y.J. Type I interferonopathies: A novel set of inborn errors of immunity. *Ann. N. Y. Acad. Sci.* **2011**, *1238*, 91–98. [CrossRef]

4. Crow, Y.J.; Black, D.N.; Ali, M.; Bond, J.; Jackson, A.P.; Lefson, M.; Michaud, J.; Roberts, E.; Stephenson, J.B.; Woods, C.G.; et al. Cree encephalitis is allelic with Aicardi-Goutiéres syndrome: Implications for the pathogenesis of disorders of interferon α metabolism. *J. Med. Genet.* **2003**, *40*, 183–187. [CrossRef] [PubMed]

5. Baechler, E.C.; Batliwalla, F.M.; Karypis, G.; Gaffney, P.M.; Ortmann, W.A.; Espe, K.J.; Shark, K.B.; Grande, W.J.; Hughes, K.M.; Kapur, V.; et al. Interferon-inducible gene expression signature in peripheral blood cells of patients with severe lupus. *Proc. Natl. Acad. Sci. USA* **2003**, *100*, 2610–2615. [CrossRef] [PubMed]

6. Rice, G.I.; Forte, G.M.; Szynkiewicz, M.; Chase, D.S.; Aeby, A.; Abdel-Hamid, M.S.; Ackroyd, S.; Allcock, R.; Bailey, K.M.; Balottin, U.; et al. Assessment of interferon-related biomarkers in Aicardi-Goutières syndrome associated with mutations in TREX1, RNASEH2A, RNASEH2B, RNASEH2C, SAMHD1, and ADAR: A case-control study. *Lancet Neurol.* **2013**, *12*, 1159–1169. [CrossRef]

7. Yao, Y.; Higgs, B.W.; Morehouse, C.; de Los Reyes, M.; Trigona, W.; Brohawn, P.; White, W.; Zhang, J.; White, B.; Coyle, A.J.; et al. Development of Potential Pharmacodynamic and Diagnostic Markers for Anti-IFN-α Monoclonal Antibody Trials in Systemic Lupus Erythematosus. *Hum. Genom. Proteom.* **2009**, *2009*. [CrossRef] [PubMed]

8. Furie, R.; Khamashta, M.; Merrill, J.T.; Werth, V.P.; Kalunian, K.; Brohawn, P.; Illei, G.G.; Drappa, J.; Wang, L.; Yoo, S.; et al. Anifrolumab, an Anti-Interferon-α Receptor Monoclonal Antibody, in Moderate-to-Severe Systemic Lupus Erythematosus. *Arthritis Rheumatol.* **2017**, *69*, 376–386. [CrossRef]

9. Merrill, J.T.; Furie, R.; Werth, V.P.; Khamashta, M.; Drappa, J.; Wang, L.; Illei, G.; Tummala, R. Anifrolumab effects on rash and arthritis: Impact of the type I interferon gene signature in the phase IIb MUSE study in patients with systemic lupus erythematosus. *Lupus Sci. Med.* **2018**, *5*, e000284. [CrossRef]

10. Rice, G.I.; Melki, I.; Frémond, M.L.; Briggs, T.A.; Rodero, M.P.; Kitabayashi, N.; Oojageer, A.; Bader-Meunier, B.; Belot, A.; Bodemer, C.; et al. Assessment of Type I Interferon Signaling in Pediatric Inflammatory Disease. *J. Clin. Immunol.* **2017**, *37*, 123–132. [CrossRef]

11. Kim, H.; Sanchez, G.A.; Goldbach-Mansky, R. Insights from Mendelian Interferonopathies: Comparison of CANDLE, SAVI with AGS, Monogenic Lupus. *J. Mol. Med.* **2016**, *94*, 1111–1127. [CrossRef] [PubMed]

12. Feng, X.; Wu, H.; Grossman, J.M.; Hanvivadhanakul, P.; FitzGerald, J.D.; Park, G.S.; Dong, X.; Chen, W.; Kim, M.H.; Weng, H.H.; et al. Association of increased interferon-inducible gene expression with disease activity and lupus nephritis in patients with systemic lupus erythematosus. *Arthritis Rheum.* **2006**, *54*, 2951–2962. [CrossRef] [PubMed]

13. Higgs, B.W.; Liu, Z.; White, B.; Zhu, W.; White, W.I.; Morehouse, C.; Brohawn, P.; Kiener, P.A.; Richman, L.; Fiorentino, D.; et al. Patients with systemic lupus erythematosus, myositis, rheumatoid arthritis and scleroderma share activation of a common type I interferon pathway. *Ann. Rheum. Dis.* **2011**, *70*, 2029–2036. [CrossRef] [PubMed]

14. Greenberg, S.A.; Pinkus, J.L.; Pinkus, G.S.; Burleson, T.; Sanoudou, D.; Tawil, R.; Barohn, R.J.; Saperstein, D.S.; Briemberg, H.R.; Ericsson, M.; et al. Interferon-α/β-mediated innate immune mechanisms in dermatomyositis. *Ann. Neurol.* **2005**, *57*, 664–678. [CrossRef] [PubMed]

15. Salajegheh, M.; Kong, S.W.; Pinkus, J.L.; Walsh, R.J.; Liao, A.; Nazareno, R.; Amato, A.A.; Krastins, B.; Morehouse, C.; Higgs, B.W.; et al. Interferon-stimulated gene 15 (ISG15) conjugates proteins in dermatomyositis muscle with perifascicular atrophy. *Ann. Neurol.* **2010**, *67*, 53–63. [CrossRef]

16. Uruha, A.; Nishikawa, A.; Tsuburaya, R.S.; Hamanaka, K.; Kuwana, M.; Watanabe, Y.; Suzuki, S.; Suzuki, N.; Nishino, I. Sarcoplasmic MxA expression: A valuable marker of dermatomyositis. *Neurology* **2017**, *88*, 493–500. [CrossRef] [PubMed]

17. Cervera, R.; Serrano, R.; Pons-Estel, G.J.; Ceberio-Hualde, L.; Shoenfeld, Y.; de Ramón, E.; Buonaiuto, V.; Jacobsen, S.; Zeher, M.M.; Tarr, T.; et al. Morbidity and mortality in the antiphospholipid syndrome during a 10-year period: A multicentre prospective study of 1000 patients. *Ann. Rheum. Dis.* **2015**, *74*, 1011–1018. [CrossRef] [PubMed]

18. Palli, E.; Kravvariti, E.; Tektonidou, M.G. Type I Interferon Signature in Primary Antiphospholipid Syndrome: Clinical and Laboratory Associations. *Front. Immunol.* **2019**, *10*, 487. [CrossRef]

19. Bernales, I.; Fullaondo, A.; Marín-Vidalled, M.J.; Ucar, E.; Martínez-Taboada, V.; López-Hoyos, M.; Zubiaga, A.M. Innate immune response gene expression profiles characterize primary antiphospholipid syndrome. *Genes Immun.* **2008**, *9*, 38–46. [CrossRef]

20. Grenn, R.C.; Yalavarthi, S.; Gandhi, A.A.; Kazzaz, N.M.; Núñez-Álvarez, C.; Hernández-Ramírez, D.; Cabral, A.R.; McCune, W.J.; Bockenstedt, P.L.; Knight, J.S. Endothelial progenitor dysfunction associates with a type I interferon signature in primary antiphospholipid syndrome. *Ann. Rheum. Dis.* **2017**, *76*, 450–457. [CrossRef]

21. van den Hoogen, L.L.; Fritsch-Stork, R.D.; Versnel, M.A.; Derksen, R.H.; van Roon, J.A.; Radstake, T.R. Monocyte type I interferon signature in antiphospholipid syndrome is related to proinflammatory monocyte subsets, hydroxychloroquine and statin use. *Ann. Rheum. Dis.* **2016**, *75*, e81. [CrossRef] [PubMed]

22. Knight, J.S.; Meng, H.; Coit, P.; Yalavarthi, S.; Sule, G.; Gandhi, A.A.; Grenn, R.C.; Mazza, L.F.; Ali, R.A.; Renauer, P.; et al. Activated signature of antiphospholipid syndrome neutrophils reveals potential therapeutic target. *JCI Insight* **2017**, *2*. [CrossRef] [PubMed]

23. Fryer, J.F.; Baylis, S.A.; Gottlieb, A.L.; Ferguson, M.; Vincini, G.A.; Bevan, V.M.; Carman, W.F.; Minor, P.D. Development of working reference materials for clinical virology. *J. Clin. Virol.* **2008**, *43*, 367–371. [CrossRef] [PubMed]

24. Kim, H.; de Jesus, A.A.; Brooks, S.R.; Liu, Y.; Huang, Y.; VanTries, R.; Montealegre Sanchez, G.A.; Rotman, Y.; Gadina, M.; Goldbach-Mansky, R. Development of a Validated Interferon Score Using NanoString Technology. *J. Interferon Cytokine Res.* **2018**, *38*, 171–185. [CrossRef] [PubMed]

25. Livak, K.J.; Schmittgen, T.D. Analysis of relative gene expression data using real-time quantitative PCR and the 2(-Delta Delta C(T)) Method. *Methods* **2001**, *25*, 402–408. [CrossRef] [PubMed]

26. Dobin, A.; Davis, C.A.; Schlesinger, F.; Drenkow, J.; Zaleski, C.; Jha, S.; Batut, P.; Chaisson, M.; Gingeras, T.R. STAR: Ultrafast universal RNA-seq aligner. *Bioinformatics* **2013**, *29*, 15–21. [CrossRef] [PubMed]

27. Liao, Y.; Smyth, G.K.; Shi, W. featureCounts: An efficient general purpose program for assigning sequence reads to genomic features. *Bioinformatics* **2014**, *30*, 923–930. [CrossRef]

28. Love, M.I.; Huber, W.; Anders, S. Moderated estimation of fold change and dispersion for RNA-seq data with DESeq2. *Genome Biol.* **2014**, *15*, 550. [CrossRef]

29. Robinson, M.D.; McCarthy, D.J.; Smyth, G.K. edgeR: A Bioconductor package for differential expression analysis of digital gene expression data. *Bioinformatics* **2010**, *26*, 139–140. [CrossRef]

30. McCarthy, D.J.; Chen, Y.; Smyth, G.K. Differential expression analysis of multifactor RNA-Seq experiments with respect to biological variation. *Nucleic Acids Res.* **2012**, *40*, 4288–4297. [CrossRef]

31. Faul, F.; Erdfelder, E.; Lang, A.G.; Buchner, A. G*Power 3: A flexible statistical power analysis program for the social, behavioral, and biomedical sciences. *Behav. Res. Methods* **2007**, *39*, 175–191. [CrossRef] [PubMed]

32. Faul, F.; Erdfelder, E.; Buchner, A.; Lang, A.G. Statistical power analyses using G*Power 3.1: Tests for correlation and regression analyses. *Behav. Res. Methods* **2009**, *41*, 1149–1160. [CrossRef] [PubMed]

33. Bodewes, I.L.A.; Björk, A.; Versnel, M.A.; Wahren-Herlenius, M. Innate immunity and interferons in the pathogenesis of Sjögren's syndrome. *Rheumatology* **2019**. [CrossRef] [PubMed]

34. Nezos, A.; Gravani, F.; Tassidou, A.; Kapsogeorgou, E.K.; Voulgarelis, M.; Koutsilieris, M.; Crow, M.K.; Mavragani, C.P. Type I and II interferon signatures in Sjogren's syndrome pathogenesis: Contributions in distinct clinical phenotypes and Sjogren's related lymphomagenesis. *J. Autoimmun.* **2015**, *63*, 47–58. [CrossRef] [PubMed]

35. Cantaert, T.; van Baarsen, L.G.; Wijbrandts, C.A.; Thurlings, R.M.; van de Sande, M.G.; Bos, C.; van der Pouw Kraan, T.C.; van der Pouw, T.K.; Verweij, C.L.; Tak, P.P.; et al. Type I interferons have no major influence on humoral autoimmunity in rheumatoid arthritis. *Rheumatology* **2010**, *49*, 156–166. [CrossRef] [PubMed]

36. Castañeda-Delgado, J.E.; Bastián-Hernandez, Y.; Macias-Segura, N.; Santiago-Algarra, D.; Castillo-Ortiz, J.D.; Alemán-Navarro, A.L.; Martínez-Tejada, P.; Enciso-Moreno, L.; Garcia-De Lira, Y.; Olguín-Calderón, D.; et al. Type I Interferon Gene Response Is Increased in Early and Established Rheumatoid Arthritis and Correlates with Autoantibody Production. *Front. Immunol.* **2017**, *8*, 285. [CrossRef]

37. Ekholm, L.; Vosslamber, S.; Tjärnlund, A.; de Jong, T.D.; Betteridge, Z.; McHugh, N.; Plestilova, L.; Klein, M.; Padyukov, L.; Voskuyl, A.E.; et al. Autoantibody Specificities and Type I Interferon Pathway Activation in Idiopathic Inflammatory Myopathies. *Scand. J. Immunol.* **2016**, *84*, 100–109. [CrossRef] [PubMed]

38. Brkic, Z.; van Bon, L.; Cossu, M.; van Helden-Meeuwsen, C.G.; Vonk, M.C.; Knaapen, H.; van den Berg, W.; Dalm, V.A.; Van Daele, P.L.; Severino, A.; et al. The interferon type I signature is present in systemic sclerosis before overt fibrosis and might contribute to its pathogenesis through high BAFF gene expression and high collagen synthesis. *Ann. Rheum. Dis.* **2016**, *75*, 1567–1573. [CrossRef] [PubMed]

39. Quartuccio, L.; Mavragani, C.P.; Nezos, A.; Gandolfo, S.; Tzioufas, A.G.; De Vita, S. Type I interferon signature may influence the effect of belimumab on immunoglobulin levels, including rheumatoid factor in Sjögren's syndrome. *Clin. Exp. Rheumatol.* **2017**, *35*, 719–720.

40. de Jong, T.D.; Vosslamber, S.; Blits, M.; Wolbink, G.; Nurmohamed, M.T.; van der Laken, C.J.; Jansen, G.; Voskuyl, A.E.; Verweij, C.L. Effect of prednisone on type I interferon signature in rheumatoid arthritis: Consequences for response prediction to rituximab. *Arthritis Res. Ther.* **2015**, *17*, 78. [CrossRef]

41. Wright, H.L.; Thomas, H.B.; Moots, R.J.; Edwards, S.W. Interferon gene expression signature in rheumatoid arthritis neutrophils correlates with a good response to TNFi therapy. *Rheumatology* **2015**, *54*, 188–193. [CrossRef] [PubMed]

42. Raterman, H.G.; Vosslamber, S.; de Ridder, S.; Nurmohamed, M.T.; Lems, W.F.; Boers, M.; van de Wiel, M.; Dijkmans, B.A.; Verweij, C.L.; Voskuyl, A.E. The interferon type I signature towards prediction of non-response to rituximab in rheumatoid arthritis patients. *Arthritis Res. Ther.* **2012**, *14*, R95. [CrossRef] [PubMed]

43. Everaert, C.; Luypaert, M.; Maag, J.L.V.; Cheng, Q.X.; Dinger, M.E.; Hellemans, J.; Mestdagh, P. Benchmarking of RNA-sequencing analysis workflows using whole-transcriptome RT-qPCR expression data. *Sci. Rep.* **2017**, *7*, 1559. [CrossRef] [PubMed]

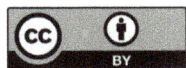

diagnostics

MDPI

Article

The HD-OCT Study May Be Useful in Searching for Markers of Preclinical Stage of Diabetic Retinopathy in Patients with Type 1 Diabetes

Magdalena Kołodziej [1], Arleta Waszczykowska [2], Irmina Korzeniewska-Dyl [3], Aleksandra Pyziak-Skupien [4], Konrad Walczak [3], Dariusz Moczulski [3], Piotr Jurowski [2], Wojciech Młynarski [5], Agnieszka Szadkowska [6] and Agnieszka Zmysłowska [6,*]

[1] Department of Practical Obstetrics, Medical University of Lodz, 90-419 Lodz, Poland
[2] Department of Ophthalmology and Vision Rehabilitation, Medical University of Lodz, 90-419 Lodz, Poland
[3] Department of Internal Medicine and Nephrodiabetology, Medical University of Lodz, 90-419 Lodz, Poland
[4] Department of Pediatrics, Silesian Medical University in Katowice, 40-055 Katowice, Poland
[5] Department of Pediatrics, Oncology and Hematology, Medical University of Lodz, 90-419 Lodz, Poland
[6] Department of Pediatrics, Diabetology, Endocrinology and Nephrology, Medical University of Lodz, 90-419 Lodz, Poland
* Correspondence: agnieszka.zmyslowska@umed.lodz.pl; Tel.: +48-42-6177750; Fax: +48-42-6177798

Received: 30 July 2019; Accepted: 23 August 2019; Published: 26 August 2019

Abstract: The aim of the study was to analyze the thickness of individual retinal layers in patients with type 1 diabetes (T1D) in comparison to the control group and in relation to markers of diabetes metabolic control. The study group consisted of 111 patients with an average of 6-years of T1D duration. The control group included 36 gender- and age-matched individuals. In all patients optical coherence tomography (OCT) study was performed using HD-OCT Cirrus 5000 with evaluation of optic nerve head (ONH) parameters, thickness of retinal nerve fiber layer (RNFL) with its quadrants, macular full-thickness parameters, ganglion cells with inner plexus layer (GCIPL) and choroidal thickness (CT). Lower disc area value was observed in the study group as compared to controls ($p = 0.0215$). Negative correlations were found both between age at examination and rim area ($R = -0.28$, $p = 0.0007$) and between superior RNFL thickness and duration of diabetes ($R = -0.20$, $p = 0.0336$). Positive correlation between center thickness and SD for average glycemia ($R = 0.30$, $p = 0.0071$) was noted. Temporal CT correlated positively with age at examination ($R = 0.21$, $p = 0.0127$). The selected parameters the HD-OCT study may in the future serve as potential markers of preclinical phase of DR in patients with T1D.

Keywords: diabetic retinopathy; type 1 diabetes; HD-OCT; ONH; RNFL; choroidal thickness

1. Introduction

Type 1 diabetes (T1D) is one of the most common metabolic diseases diagnosed in children and is associated with the risk of development of numerous chronic complications. Diabetic eye disease—as the most common of the chronic complications of T1D—may be connected with abnormalities in various eye structures. However, the complication related to the greatest risk of loss of vision is diabetic retinopathy (DR) and accompanying diabetic macular edema (DME) [1,2]. DR is considered to be the earliest chronic complication of type 1 diabetes because it is present even after several years of its course [3]. The development and progression of diabetic retinopathy is influenced mainly by the degree of metabolic diabetes control, diabetes duration, presence of dyslipidemia, proteinuria, arterial hypertension, pregnancy and genetic predisposition [4]. Many studies have shown that proper control of glycemia, blood pressure and lipid levels may reduce the risk of DR development and significantly slow its progression [5].

Currently, fluorescein angiography (FA) remains the gold standard in the diagnosis of clinical phase of diabetic retinopathy, which enables detailed assessment of blood vessels of the fundus of the eye as an invasive method [6]. FA is a test that involves taking a series of photographs of the fundus after intravenous administration of a contrast agent (fluorescein). FA enables visualization of the circulation in the retinal vessels and indirectly the uvea, as well as evaluation of the state of the retinal pigment epithelium and retinal blood vessels which are not visible during fundus examination. This technique has become fundamental when assessing the complications of diabetic retinopathy, retinal vascular obstruction, or when diagnosing many macular diseases. However, FA is associated with severe potential risks [7].

Thus, in an attempt to optimize diagnostic procedures, the most informative and least invasive diagnostic method should be identified. Optical coherence tomography (OCT) is a safe, non-contact, non-invasive and effective technique of imaging tissue and could be considered as a valid alternative to FA. Intra-retinal leakage is not necessary to confirm the presence of DME, and FA is useful only as a guide for focal or grid laser treatment of thickened areas. Therefore, numerous new diagnostic tools such as high-definition OCT (HD-OCT) and spectral-domain (SD) OCT are being evaluated clinically. These methods provide improved capabilities for the imaging of the intra-retinal morphology and/or allow for the analysis of the structural and functional aspects of leakage activity. Moreover, they offer realistic 3D imaging of retinal and subretinal levels in various diseases [8]. Cirrus HD-OCT (Carl Zeiss Meditec, Inc., Dublin, OH, USA) is an SD-OCT that has an axial resolution of 5 μm and a scan velocity of 27,000 axial scans per second. These features improve the ability to visualize smaller and thinner structures that are difficult to visualize with time-domain OCT (Stratus OCT).

Therefore, alternative imaging methods such as OCT study are suggested in patients, especially considering the new approach to pathologic mechanisms leading to DR development [9]. Until now, diabetic retinopathy has been considered to be a mainly vascular complication, however, it is now known that neurodegenerative processes take place in the retina before the clinical retinopathy, which is its preclinical period [5]. Recent publications have shown that these early symptoms of neuronal damage of the retinal layer are present before the appearance of changes visible at the fundus of the eye and may contribute to the development of microvascular abnormalities [10,11]. These reports also indicate a decrease in retinal thickness in diabetic patients, mainly in macular ganglion cells. This suggests progress in neurodegeneration as an early, preclinical stage of diabetic retinopathy [12,13].

In addition, it is known that previous attempts to treat diabetic retinopathy are being made in its clinical phase [14,15], whereas, from the patient's point of view, it would be worthwhile to try to stop the progress of retinal neurodegeneration at the earliest possible stage [16]. The lack of unambiguously defined early markers of DR preclinical phase leads to their search based on new and non-invasive imaging studies.

The aim of the study was to evaluate the thickness of retina in its individual layers in patients with type 1 diabetes as compared to the control group and in relation to the parameters of metabolic diabetes control.

2. Materials and Methods

The study was conducted in accordance with the Declaration of Helsinki, and the study protocol was approved by the University Bioethics Committee at the Medical University in Lodz, Poland (RNN/374/17/KE, 19/12/2017). Patients and/or their parents gave written informed consent for participation in the study.

The work described has been carried out in accordance with The Declaration of Helsinki of 1975 and revised in 2013 for experiments involving humans.

The study group consisted of 111 patients (F-61/M-50) including 82 children and 29 adults aged 5.6 to 50.8 (min-max) years at the time of study, with an average 6-year course of clinically overt T1D. In all patients, diabetes was diagnosed according to WHO criteria. The presence of autoantibodies characteristic for T1D and decreased C-peptide plasma levels were observed in all patients at T1D onset. Detailed characteristics of the study group are shown in Table 1.

Table 1. Characteristics of the study group of patients with type 1 diabetes (T1D).

Parameter	Median or Percentage	IQR–Interquartile Range
Age at T1D onset (years)	8.63	4.5–10.8
Diabetes duration (years)	6.02	3.9–10.2
Age at examination (years)	14.47	10.7–20.6
Gender (F/M; %)	55/45	-
Average HbA1c level (%/mmol/mol)	7.10/54.1	6.7/49.77–8/63.9
Average blood glucose level (mg/dL)	155	135–180
Standard deviation for blood glucose level	72	59–79
BMI-Z-score at examination	0.55	−0.36–1.12
Insulin uptake (U/kg)	0.80	0.60–1.07
Total cholesterol (mg/dL)	181.53	153–311
LDL-cholesterol (mg/dL)	110	87–211
HDL-cholesterol (mg/dL)	62	52–98
Triglycerides (mg/dL)	75	55–110
Serum creatinine level (mg/dL)	0.66	0.6–0.7

The control group consisted of 36 healthy (F-23/M-13) gender- ($p = 0.3466$) and age-matched ($p = 0.1688$) individuals with no glucose tolerance disturbances.

Patients under 5 years of age with diagnosed arterial hypertension, clinically manifest diabetic retinopathy, diabetic kidney disease and previous ocular surgery, any eye disease, myopia and hyperopia above 3 diopters, chronic use of topical medications were excluded from the study and control groups.

The HD-OCT study was performed in the patients from the study and control groups in the Department of Ophthalmology and Vision Rehabilitation of the Medical University of Lodz, Poland using the Cirrus HD-OCT device (5000: Carl Zeiss Meditec. Inc., Dublin, OH, USA) after mydriasis and evaluated independently by two experienced ophthalmologists.

Two scans, including one macular scan centered on the fovea (macular cube 512 × 128 protocol) and one peripapillary retinal nerve fiber layer (RNFL) scan centered on the optic disc (optic disc cube 200 × 200 protocol) were acquired through dilated pupils. The mean retinal thickness values were obtained on all images for foveal subfield and the inner and outer rings of a standard ETDRS (Early Treatment of Diabetic Retinopathy Study) grid. Macular ganglion cell layer/inner plexiform layer (GCIPL), RNFL (retinal nerve fiber layer) and optic nerve head (ONH) parameters were measured automatically using the internal ganglion cell, RNFL and ONH analysis algorithms, respectively. The following GCIPL thickness measurements were analyzed: Average, minimum and sectoral (superonasal, superior, superotemporal, inferotemporal, inferior and inferonasal). RNFL total thickness as well as superior, inferior, temporal and nasal RNFL thickness were evaluated. For the ONH analysis, the following parameters were included: Disc area, rim area, cup volume and cup-to-disc (c/d) ratio. Choroidal thickness (CT) was measured manually from the outer portion of the hyperreflective line corresponding to the retinal pigment epithelium to the inner surface of the sclera, using the Cirrus linear measurement tool (HD 21-line raster). To be included in this study, images had to be at least 6 of 10 in intensity and taken as close to the fovea as possible, by choosing to image the thinnest point of the macula, with the understanding that slight differences in positioning could affect the measured thickness. Choroidal thickness was measured at the fovea and 1-mm temporal and nasal to the fovea. Averages from measurements in both eyes were calculated and used for further analysis.

The HD-OCT results were related to individual parameters and indicators of clinical course of diabetes including: Age at the time of the study (years), gender, age at diabetes onset (years), duration of diabetes (years), average HbA1c from the last year preceding the study (%), average blood glucose (BG) level from 14 days before an examination (mg/dL), standard deviation (SD) for BG evaluating the fluctuations in BG results from 14 days before an examination, BMI-Z-score and mean insulin uptake (U/kg).

HbA1c was determined by high-performance liquid chromatography (HPLC) using the Bio-Rad VARIANT™ Hemoglobin A1c Program (Bio-Rad Laboratories Inc., Hercules, CA, USA) with its values represented as percentages and in addition as mmol/mol according to IFCC (International Federation of Clinical Chemistry).

Statistical Analysis

The assessment of the normality of distribution was carried out using the Kolmogorov-Smirnov test and verified by the Shapiro-Wilk test. Comparisons of the HD-OCT variables between study and control groups were performed using a non-parametric Mann-Whitney's test. For the correlation analysis, a Spearman correlation test was used. Categorical variables were presented as numbers with appropriate percentages and continuous variables as medians with interquartile range (IQR). Results with p-values < 0.05 were considered as statistically significant. Analyses were performed using Statistica 13.1 PL software (Statsoft, Tulsa, OK, USA).

3. Results

The parameters of optic nerve head (ONH); thickness of retinal nerve fiber layer (RNFL) and its quadrants; average retinal thickness, central retinal thickness, total retinal volume; macular ganglion cell layer/inner plexiform layer (GCIPL) thickness; and choroidal thickness (CT) were compared between the study and control groups. A significantly lower disc area value was observed in the study group (Me 1.84 mm^2; IQR 1.62–2.04) in comparison to the control group (Me 1.98 mm^2; IQR 1.82–2.14, p = 0.0215) (Table 2). There were no statistically significant differences in other HD–OCT parameters between the studied groups (Table 2).

Table 2. Comparison of the parameters of ONH, thickness of RNFL and its quadrants, average retinal thickness, central retinal thickness, total retinal volume, CT and GCIPL thickness, assessed using high-definition optical coherence tomography HD-OCT of the study group of patients with T1D and control group.

Parameter	Study Group Median (IQR)	Control Group Median (IQR)	p Level
Disc area (mm^2)	**1.84 (1.62–2.04)**	**1.98 (1.82–2.14)**	**0.0214**
Rim area (mm^2)	1.43 (1.28–1.63)	1.53 (1.31–1.71)	0.2553
c/d area ratio	0.42 (0.33–0.55)	0.45 (0.32–0.56)	0.6356
Vertical CDR	0.41 (0.32–0.52)	0.43 (0.29–0.53)	0.8136
Cup volume (mm^3)	0.07 (0.02–0.16)	0.08 (0.03–0.22)	0.4646
RNFL Total Thickness (μm)	93.00 (86.00–101.50)	91.25 (87.50–98.51)	0.4640
Superior RNFL thickness (μm)	116.50 (108.50–128.50)	117.50 (107.00–127.50)	0.6884
Inferior RNFL thickness (μm)	124.50 (109.50–134.50)	122.00 (113.25–128.75)	0.5841
Temporal RNFL thickness (μm)	63.50 (57.50–70.50)	63.75 (55.25–71.00)	0.8605
Nasal RNFL thickness (μm)	69.50 (60.50–76.50)	70.00 (60.5–74.00)	0.6686
Macular average thickness (μm)	283.50 (274.50–293.50)	284.25 (276.25–294.75)	0.4401
Center thickness (μm)	253.25 (241.00–264.00)	255.50 (240.75–266.00)	0.6661
Total macular volume (mm^3)	10.20 (9.85–10.55)	10.22 (9.95–10.60)	0.3400
Choroidal thickness subfoveal (μm)	352.00 (319.50–393.00)	360.75 (331.50–399.75)	0.3528
Choroidal thickness nasal (μm)	354.00 (318.50–389.00)	359.00 (326.25–376.50)	0.8965
Choroidal thickness temporal (μm)	336.50 (301.50–384.50)	352.75 (314.50–383.00)	0.3070
Average GCLIPL thickness (μm)	83.50 (79.50–88.00)	82.25 (78.75–86.75)	0.6005
Minimum GCLIPL thickness (μm)	81.50 (76.50–86.00)	80.50 (76.75–83.75)	0.7340
GCLIPL superior (μm)	83.50 (79.00–87.50)	82.50 (77.75–87.00)	0.2140
GCLIPL superior-nasal (μm)	85.00 (81.50–89.50)	83.00 (79.50–87.00)	0.1240
GCLIPL inferior-nasal (μm)	84.00 (79.50–88.50)	81.75 (78.00–86.00)	0.1551
GCLIPL inferior (μm)	82.00 (78.00–86.00)	80.75 (77.50–86.00)	0.7551
GCLIPL inferior-temporal (μm)	83.50 (80.00–88.50)	82.75 (78.25–86.25)	0.3227
GCLIPL superior-temporal (μm)	82.50 (78.52–86.50)	81.50 (77.00–84.50)	0.2982

T1D—type 1 diabetes, IQR—interquartile range, ONH—optic nerve head, RNFL—retinal nerve fiber layer, GCILP—ganglion cell layer/inner plexiform layer, CT—choroidal thickness; p < 0.05 are indicated in bold.

Then, in the study group the correlations between HD-OCT and individual parameters and markers of clinical course of diabetes were analyzed.

A negative correlation between rim area and age at the time of examination was observed (R = −0.28, *p* = 0.0007) (Figure 1). Moreover, the c/d ratio correlated positively with age of patients at the study time (R = 0.17, *p* = 0.0449). There was also a tendency to negative correlations between rim area and age at T1D onset (R = −0.19, *p* = 0.0517) and disc area and HbA1c value (R = −0.17, *p* = 0.0843).

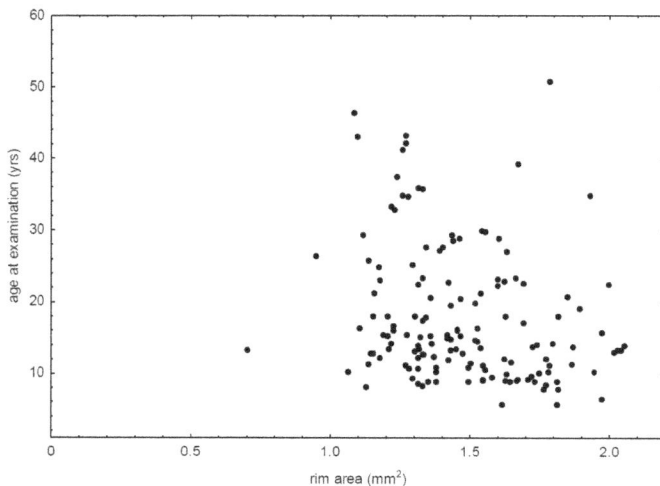

Figure 1. Correlation between rim area and age at examination in patients with type 1 diabetes (R = −0.28, *p* = 0.0007).

In the study group, negative correlations between superior RNFL thickness and duration of diabetes (R = −0.20, *p* = 0.0336) (Figure 2) and between inferior RNFL thickness and HbA1c (R = −0.20, *p* = 0.0364) were also noted. There were positive correlations between macular center thickness and SD for average blood glucose level (R = 0.30, *p* = 0.0071).

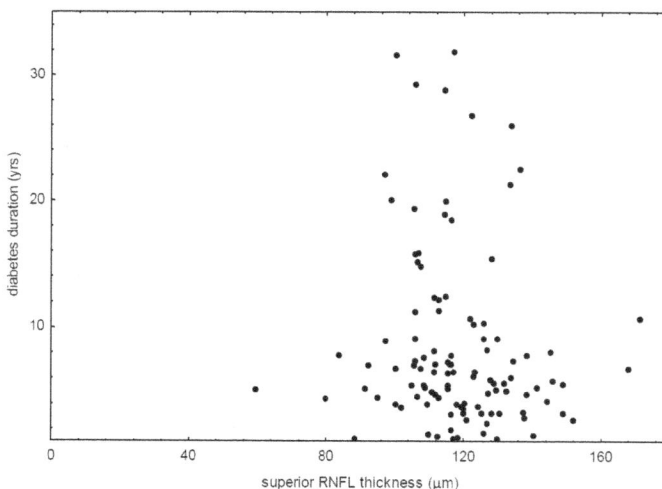

Figure 2. Correlation between thickness of superior retinal nerve fiber layer and duration of type 1 diabetes (R = −0.20, *p* = 0.0336).

The age of patients at the study time showed a trend to negative correlations with both average GCIPL thickness (R = −0.15, p = 0.0706) and GCIPL lower thickness (R = −0.15, p = 0.0759). A trend with respect to a negative correlation between GCIPL low-temporal thickness and HbA1c (R = −0.18, p = 0.0696) was also found.

It was also observed that temporal CT correlated positively both with age at the examination time (R = 0.21, p = 0.0127) (Figure 3) and age at diabetes diagnosis (R = 0.22, p = 0.0255). A positive correlation was also found between the subfoveal CT and the age at diabetes onset (R = 0.23, p = 0.0189), while a tendency to a positive correlation between the subfoveal CT and the age at examination (R = 0.16, p = 0.0596) was observed. Other parameters of clinical course of type 1 diabetes did not correlate with the HD-OCT parameters (p > 0.1).

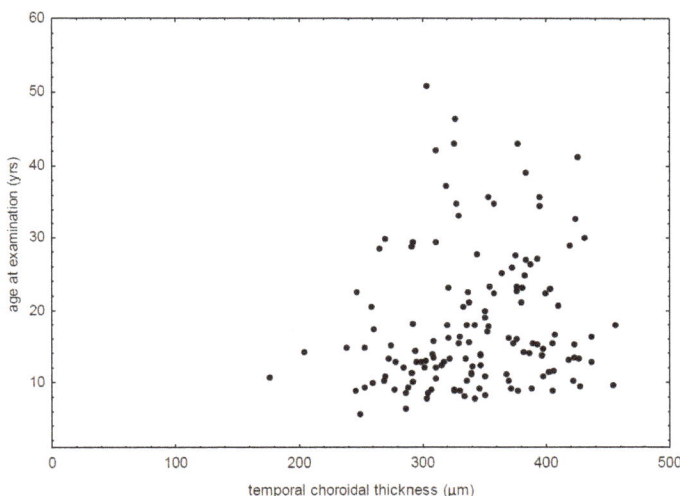

Figure 3. Correlation between temporal choroidal thickness and age at examination in patients with type 1 diabetes (R = 0.21, p = 0.0127).

4. Discussion

In the present study, for the first time such a large number of patients with type 1 diabetes, both children and young adults, were examined using the HD-OCT study.

A significant reduction of the disc area in the study group was observed in comparison to healthy controls. Moreover, in patients with T1D the selected ONH parameters correlated with their age. In previous studies, no differences in rim area, disc area or cup to disc ratio between pediatric patients with T1D and control group [17] were found. Only significant differences in c/d ratio were noted in patients with type 2 diabetes (T2D) without DR as compared to the control group [18]. In the studies, more binocular RNFL thickness asymmetry in diabetic patients in relation to the controls without significant differences in RNFL thickness [17,18] was also noted.

In our study, negative correlations in the study group between superior RNFL thickness and duration of diabetes, and between inferior RNFL thickness and mean HbA1c value were observed. Similar to our results, Tekin et al. noticed negative correlations between both global RNFL thickness and macular thickness and HbA1c value and diabetes duration using the SD-OCT study in children with T1D without clinical overt DR. They also found significantly thinner global RNFL thickness as well as temporal and inferior outer macular thickness in relation to the controls [19]. Both overall and superior RNFL thickness correlated with the age of T1D patients in the Dehghani et al. study, at the same time being an indicator of peripheral neuropathy in the patients [20]. In other research, the significant thinning of RNFL and its individual quadrants was confirmed in T2D patients without retinopathy in comparison to the controls [21]. Furthermore, there are also studies in which RNFL thinning was found to correlate with the severity of retinopathy, but it was found also in T2D patients [22]. Interestingly, early structural damage of neuroretina was also related to glucose fluctuations assessed in continuous glucose monitoring (CGM) in the group of T1D patients [23]. In our study, to evaluate glucose variability, the SD for the average blood glucose (BG) level was measured within the two weeks prior to the HD-OCT study. However, it correlated positively only with macular center thickness confirming earlier reports of the effect of glucose fluctuations on the DR presence accompanied by DME [24,25].

In the present study, no differences were found between the groups with respect to other macular full-thickness parameters or GCIPL thickness. Only tendencies to correlation of average GCIPL and lower GCIPL thickness with age and HbA1c were observed. In several studies, however, a reduced GCIPL thickness was found in both pediatric T1D patients and adults with T2D without retinopathy, suggesting that the presence of chronic hyperglycemia may have an early neurodegenerative effect on retinal ganglion cells, even when vascular disorders are not yet present [26,27].

Previous studies on DR pathogenesis have shown that neuronal dysfunction and progressive neurodegeneration are closely correlated with microvascular disorders. According to many authors, the best method to prevent the appearance of diabetic eye disease is correct glycemic control, reducing the risk of developing microvascular complications [28]. However, it seems that local hyperperfusion may be present already at the preclinical stage of DR and may accompany the neurodegeneration progress. In the paper by Golebiewska et al. it was noted that—besides the presence of early neuroretinal lesions—the central choroidal thickness tends to be thicker in T1D children without DR in comparison to healthy children and shows a correlation with gender of the subjects in favor of girls. However, it does not correlate with the duration of diabetes or HbA1c [29]. In our study we did not observe a relationship between CT and the gender, but with the age of the subjects. Moreover, positive correlations between subfoveal and temporal parts of CT with the age of patients were found, both at the time of examination and at the time of diabetes diagnosis.

The Niestrata-Ortiz et al. study carried out in the group of children with type 1 diabetes compared to the age-matched control group also revealed that choroidal thickness is higher in patients with T1D compared to the control group, and increases with the duration of diabetes, which makes it useful for screening in children with type 1 diabetes [30].

Concluding, the results obtained in the group of children and young adults with type 1 diabetes indicate a relationship between age of patients, duration of diabetes, chronic hyperglycemia, glycemia fluctuations and the size of the ONH parameters, thickness of superior and inferior RNFL quadrant, center macular thickness and subfoveal and temporal choroidal thickness.

Our findings can also confirm earlier observations of the researchers that the Cirrus HD-OCT system achieves approximately double the axial resolution of the previous generation Stratus OCT device and allows for better visualization of tissues. This processing HD-OCT software is unique because images are generated by evaluating all of the pixel data to reduce noise and construct the best possible image. This enables visualization and measurement of the full thickness of the choroid and satisfactory repeatable GCIPL thickness measurements using the Cirrus HD-OCT Ganglion Cell Analysis (GCA) algorithm [31,32].

The limitation of our work may be the lack of other—apart from SD for blood glucose level—indicators of glycemia variability, which require CGM system connection to patients, as well as ophthalmic parameters, including the assessment of visual acuity. The obtained results also require further confirmation on a larger group of patients.

However, it seems that simultaneous measurement of choroidal thickness and several neurodegeneration parameters using HD-OCT is useful and the selected parameters may be promising markers of preclinical phase of diabetic retinopathy in patients with type 1 diabetes. This indicates the usefulness of the HD-OCT study as a diagnostic tool and confirms the need for the HD-OCT study in patients with several years of clinical course of type 1 diabetes.

Author Contributions: Conceptualization, A.Z. and W.M.; methodology, A.W., M.K. and P.J.; software, A.P.-S.; investigation, I.K.-D., K.W., D.M. and A.S.Z.; writing—original draft preparation, M.K.; writing—review and editing, A.Z.

Funding: This research received no external funding.

Conflicts of Interest: The authors declare no conflict of interest.

References

1. Barber, A.J. A new view of diabetic retinopathy: A neurodegenerative disease of the eye. *Prog. Neuropsychopharmacol. Biol. Psychiatry* **2003**, *27*, 283–290. [CrossRef]
2. Lechner, J.; O'Leary, O.E.; Stitt, A.W. The pathology associated with diabetic retinopathy. *Vis. Res.* **2017**, *139*, 7–14.
3. Song, S.H. Significant retinopathy in young-onset type 2 vs. type 1 diabetes: A clinical observation. *Int. J. Clin. Pract.* **2016**, *70*, 853–860. [CrossRef] [PubMed]
4. Cunha-Vaz, J.; Ribeiro, L.; Lobo, C. Phenotypes and biomarkers of diabetic retinopathy. *Prog. Retin. Eye Res.* **2014**, *41*, 90–111. [CrossRef] [PubMed]
5. Matuszewski, W.; Bandurska-Stankiewicz, E.; Modzelewski, R.; Kamińska, U.; Stefanowicz-Rutkowska, M. Diagnosis and treatment of diabetic retinopathy—Historical overview. *Clin. Diabetol.* **2017**, *6*, 182–188. [CrossRef]
6. Sosenko, J.M.; Skyler, J.S.; Mahon, J.; Krischer, J.P.; Greenbaum, C.J.; Rafkin, L.E.; Beam, C.A.; Boulware, D.C.; Matheson, D.; Cuthbertson, D.; et al. Type 1 Diabetes TrialNet and Diabetes Prevention Trial-Type 1 Study Groups. Use of the Diabetes Prevention Trial-Type 1 Risk Score (DPTRS) for improving the accuracy of the risk classification of type 1 diabetes. *Diabetes Care* **2014**, *37*, 979–984. [CrossRef]
7. Gallego-Pinazo, R.; Suelves-Cogollos, A.M.; Dolz-Marco, R.; Arevalo, J.F.; García-Delpech, S.; Mullor, J.L.; Díaz-Llopis, M. Macular laser photocoagulation guided by spectral-domain optical coherence tomography versus fluorescein angiography for diabetic macular edema. *Clin. Ophthalmol.* **2011**, *5*, 613–617.
8. Malamos, P.; Sacu, S.; Georgopoulos, M.; Kiss, C.; Pruente, C.; Schmidt-Erfurth, U. Correlation of high-definition optical coherence tomography and fluorescein angiography imagining in neovascular macular degeneration. *Invest. Ophthalmol. Vis. Sci.* **2009**, *10*, 4926–4933. [CrossRef]
9. Khadamy, J.; Abri Aghdam, K.; Falavarjani, K.G. An Update on Optical Coherence Tomography Angiography in Diabetic Retinopathy. *J. Ophthalmic Vis. Res.* **2018**, *13*, 487–497.
10. Santos, A.R.; Ribeiro, L.; Bandello, F.; Lattanzio, R.; Egan, C.; Frydkjaer-Olsen, U.; García-Arumí, J.; Gibson, J.; Grauslund, J.; Harding, S.P.; et al. European Consortium for the Early Treatment of Diabetic Retinopathy (EUROCONDOR). Functional and Structural Findings of Neurodegeneration in Early Stages of Diabetic Retinopathy: Cross-sectional Analyses of Baseline Data of the EUROCONDOR Project. *Diabetes* **2017**, *66*, 2503–2510. [CrossRef]
11. Arroba, A.I.; Mazzeo, A.; Cazzoni, D.; Beltramo, E.; Hernández, C.; Porta, M.; Simó, R.; Valverde, Á.M. Somatostatin protects photoreceptor cells against high glucose-induced apoptosis. *Mol. Vis.* **2016**, *22*, 1522–1531.
12. Gonul, S.; Ozkagnici, A.; Kerimoglu, H.; Öztürk, B.T.; Sahin, A. Evaluation of retinal nerve fiber layer thickness with optical coherence tomography in type 1 diabetes mellitus patients. Turkiye Klinikleri. *J. Med. Sci.* **2011**, *31*, 1100–1105.
13. Vujosevic, S.; Midena, E. Retinal Layers Changes in Human Preclinical and Early Clinical Diabetic Retinopathy Support Early Retinal Neuronal and Müller Cells Alterations. *J. Diabetes Res.* **2013**, 905058. [CrossRef]
14. Bressler, S.B.; Qin, H.; Beck, R.W.; Chalam, K.V.; Kim, J.E.; Melia, M.; Wells, J.A., 3rd. Diabetic Retinopathy Clinical Research Network. Factors associated with changes in visual acuity and central subfield thickness at 1 year after treatment for diabetic macular edema with ranibizumab. *Arch. Ophthalmol.* **2012**, *130*, 1153–1161. [CrossRef]
15. Do, D.V.; Nguyen, Q.D.; Boyer, D.; Schmidt-Erfurth, U.; Brown, D.M.; Vitti, R.; Berliner, A.J.; Gao, B.; Zeitz, O.; Ruckert, R.; et al. One-year out- comes of the DA VINCI Study of VEGF Trap-Eye in eyes with diabetic macular edema. *Ophthalmology* **2012**, *119*, 1658–1665. [CrossRef]

16. Hernández, C.; Bogdanov, P.; Solà-Adell, C.; Sampedro, J.; Valeri, M.; Genís, X.; Simó-Servat, O.; García-Ramírez, M.; Simó, R. Topical administration of DPP-IV inhibitors prevents retinal neurodegeneration in experimental diabetes. *Diabetologia* **2017**, *60*, 2285–2298. [CrossRef]

17. Pekel, E.; Altıncık, S.A.; Pekel, G. Evaluation of optic disc, retinal nerve fiber and macular ganglion cell layers in pediatric diabetes. *Int. Ophthalmol.* **2018**, *38*, 1955–1961. [CrossRef]

18. Pekel, E.; Tufaner, G.; Kaya, H.; Kaşikçi, A.; Deda, G.; Pekel, G. Assessment of optic disc and ganglion cell layer in diabetes mellitus type 2. *Medicine* **2017**, *96*, e7556. [CrossRef]

19. Tekin, K.; Inanc, M.; Kurnaz, E.; Bayramoglu, E.; Aydemir, E.; Koc, M.; Kiziltoprak, H.; Aycan, Z. Quantitative evaluation of early retinal changes in children with type 1 diabetes mellitus without retinopathy. *Clin. Exp. Optom.* **2018**, *101*, 680–685. [CrossRef]

20. Dehghani, C.; Srinivasan, S.; Edwards, K.; Pritchard, N.; Russell, A.W.; Malik, R.A.; Efron, N. Presence of Peripheral Neuropathy Is Associated with Progressive Thinning of Retinal Nerve Fiber Layer in Type 1 Diabetes. *Investig. Ophthalmol. Vis. Sci.* **2017**, *58*, 234–239. [CrossRef]

21. Mehboob, M.A.; Amin, Z.A.; Islam, O.U. Comparison of retinal nerve fiber layer thickness between normal population and patients with diabetes mellitus using optical coherence tomography. *Pak. J. Med. Sci.* **2019**, *35*, 29–33. [CrossRef]

22. Nadri, G.; Saxena, S.; Stefanickova, J.; Ziak, P.; Benacka, J.; Gilhotra, J.S.; Kruzliak, P. Disorganization of retinal inner layers correlates with ellipsoid zone disruption and retinal nerve fiber layer thinning in diabetic retinopathy. *J. Diabetes Complicat.* **2019**, *33*, 550–553. [CrossRef]

23. Picconi, F.; Parravano, M.; Ylli, D.; Pasqualetti, P.; Coluzzi, S.; Giordani, I.; Malandrucco, I.; Lauro, D.; Scarinci, F.; Giorno, P.; et al. Retinal neurodegeneration in patients with type 1 diabetes mellitus: The role of glycemic variability. *Acta Diabetol.* **2017**, *54*, 489–497. [CrossRef]

24. Sartore, G.; Chilelli, N.C.; Burlina, S.; Lapolla, A. Association between glucose variability as assessed by continuous glucose monitoring (CGM) and diabetic retinopathy in type 1 and type 2 diabetes. *Acta Diabetol.* **2013**, *50*, 437–442. [CrossRef]

25. Chatziralli, I.P. The Role of Glycemic Control and Variability in Diabetic Retinopathy. *Diabetes Ther.* **2018**, *9*, 431–434. [CrossRef]

26. Li, S.T.; Wang, X.N.; Du, X.H.; Wu, Q. Comparison of spectral-domain optical coherence tomography for intra-retinal layers thickness measurements between healthy and diabetic eyes among Chinese adults. *PLoS ONE* **2017**, *12*, e0177515. [CrossRef]

27. Karti, O.; Nalbantoglu, O.; Abali, S.; Ayhan, Z.; Tunc, S.; Kusbeci, T.; Ozkan, B. Retinal Ganglion Cell Loss in Children with Type 1 Diabetes Mellitus without Diabetic Retinopathy. *Ophthalmic Surg. Lasers Imaging Retina* **2017**, *48*, 473–477. [CrossRef]

28. Kase, S.; Endo, H.; Takahashi, M.; Saito, M.; Yokoi, M.; Ito, Y.; Katsuta, S.; Sonoda, S.; Sakamoto, T.; Ishida, S.; et al. Alteration of choroidal vascular structure in diabetic retinopathy. *Br. J. Ophthalmol.* **2019**. [CrossRef]

29. Gołębiewska, J.; Olechowski, A.; Wysocka-Mincewicz, M.; Baszyńska-Wilk, M.; Groszek, A.; Czeszyk-Piotrowicz, A.; Szalecki, M.; Hautz, W. Choroidal Thickness and Ganglion Cell Complex in Pubescent Children with Type 1 Diabetes without Diabetic Retinopathy Analyzed by Spectral Domain Optical Coherence Tomography. *J. Diabetes Res.* **2018**, *2018*, 5458015.

30. Niestrata-Ortiz, M.; Fichna, P.; Stankiewicz, W.; Stopa, M. Determining the effect of diabetes duration on retinal and choroidal thicknesses in children with type 1 diabetes mellitus. *Retina* **2018**. [CrossRef]

31. Manjunath, V.; Taha, M.; Fujimoto, J.G.; Duker, J.S. Choroidal Thickness in Normal Eyes Measured Using Cirrus-HD Optical Coherence Tomography. *Am. J. Ophthalmol.* **2010**, *150*, 325–329. [CrossRef]

32. Lee, S.Y.; Jeoung, J.W.; Park, K.H.; Kim, D.M. Macular ganglion cell imaging study: Interocular symmetry of ganglion cell-inner plexiform layer thickness in normal healthy eyes. *Am. J. Ophthalmol.* **2015**, *159*, 315–323. [CrossRef]

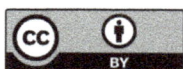

Review

Current Diabetes Technology: Striving for the Artificial Pancreas

Natalie Allen * and Anshu Gupta

Division of Pediatric Endocrinology, Virginia Commonwealth University, Children's Hospital of Richmond, Richmond, VA 23298, USA; anshu.gupta@vcuhealth.org
* Correspondence: natalie.allen@vcuhealth.org

Received: 6 February 2019; Accepted: 12 March 2019; Published: 15 March 2019

Abstract: Diabetes technology has continually evolved over the years to improve quality of life and ease of care for affected patients. Frequent blood glucose (BG) checks and multiple daily insulin injections have become standard of care in Type 1 diabetes (T1DM) management. Continuous glucose monitors (CGM) allow patients to observe and discern trends in their glycemic control. These devices improve quality of life for parents and caregivers with preset alerts for hypoglycemia. Insulin pumps have continued to improve and innovate since their emergence into the market. Hybrid closed-loop systems have harnessed the data gathered with CGM use to aid in basal insulin dosing and hypoglycemia prevention. As technology continues to progress, patients will likely have to enter less and less information into their pump system manually. In the future, we will likely see a system that requires no manual patient input and allows users to eat throughout the day without counting carbohydrates or entering in any blood sugars. As technology continues to advance, endocrinologists and diabetes providers need to stay current to better guide their patients in optimal use of emerging management tools.

Keywords: type 1 diabetes; continuous glucose monitor; insulin pump; continuous insulin infusion system; hybrid closed-loop system; diabetes technology

1. Introduction

Type 1 diabetes (T1DM) is an autoimmune disease in which the β cells of the pancreas are damaged and subsequently destroyed. Since these cells are critical in the production of insulin hormone, this leads to a state of insulin deficiency. Landmark studies, such as the Diabetes Control and Complications Trial (DCCT) and the ongoing Epidemiology of Diabetes Interventions and Complications (EDIC) follow up study, have conclusively proven the long-term benefits of early and intensive blood glucose control on the future development of diabetes-related complications, such as heart, eye, kidney, and nerve disease, and improved life expectancy [1]. As a result, frequent blood glucose (BG) checks and multiple daily insulin injections have become standard of care in T1DM management. These advances have brought forth challenges of managing a chronic illness as well as opportunities to apply technological advances from engineering to medicine.

Diabetes was referenced as early as 1500 B.C. in Egyptian manuscripts as a disease noted for increased urination. The techniques for diagnosis of T1DM were described by the middle of the 16th century when it was recognized by detection of sugar in the urine [2]. However, insulin was not discovered until 1921, when Charles Best and Frederick Banting used canine pancreas extracts to successfully treat diabetic dogs. In 1923, Eli Lilly introduced the first insulin product, a further purified pancreas extract, to the market [3]. Since that time, many different insulins and innovative insulin delivery devices have been developed from insulin pens to insulin pumps. Both diagnostic tools and treatments have continued to evolve in the 20th and 21st centuries.

The field of glucose monitoring and insulin administration technology has transformed in the past two decades. Patients in the developed world use palm-size or smaller handheld glucometers as a standard of care for managing their diabetes. Additionally, continuous glucose monitor (CGM) devices, which allow patients to wear a sensor and obtain frequent automated BG readings, are quickly gaining a central place in T1DM management. Furthermore, integrated insulin pump and CGM systems are now increasingly available; this has improved the ease of insulin delivery in addition to prevention of severe hypoglycemia, one of the most feared complications of treatment with insulin. As the technology in diabetes care continues to evolve, providers must be up-to-date on available systems and advocate for the care of their patients. In this review article, we discuss currently available and shortly anticipated diabetes technology available for T1DM patients within the United States (US) and Europe with the goal of providing a historical perspective and an update to clinicians caring for patients with diabetes so they can facilitate discussions on therapeutic options with their patients.

2. Methods

A thorough review of the existing literature was conducted via PubMed and Google Scholar. Keywords included were 'diabetes', 'T1DM', 'continuous glucose monitor', 'CGM', 'insulin pump', 'continuous insulin infusion system', 'hybrid closed loop system', 'bihormonal', 'Abbott Freestyle Libre', 'Dexcom', 'Medtronic', 'Tandem', 'OmniPod', 'iLet'. Relevant studies from 2007–2019 published in the English language were reviewed and included.

3. Continuous Glucose Monitors

Continuous glucose monitors are devices that help patients with diabetes to monitor their glucose levels over time. They allow for dynamic information that indicates direction of glucose change allowing the user to observe the influence of diet, exercise, and insulin dosing on the patient's glucose level in real-time. Additionally, they can be used in conjunction with insulin pumps to better guide insulin therapy. Studies have shown that CGM use can increase time spent in normoglycemia and decrease the frequency and severity of hypoglycemia episodes [4,5]. In a randomized study of adults with hypoglycemia unawareness, researchers found that patients in the CGM group had a 72% reduction in hypoglycemia events [6]. Alarms may be set on some of these devices to alert the user to urgent low glucose levels or elevated glucose levels. Many devices even allow sharing of data to multiple smartphones providing parents with access to remotely monitor their child's glucose levels and allowing physicians to view their patient's glucose trends and accordingly adjust insulin therapy [7].

Medtronic Minimed CGM was the first CGM system approved by the FDA in 1999 after it had been tested in Caucasian adults with T1DM [8]. This first available system was not meant to be used in real-time and BG trends could only be evaluated after the window of therapy [9]. Additionally, the FDA specifically stipulated that this device be used in conjunction with regular finger-stick BG checks. Over the 20 years since the introduction of the first CGM system to market, many new systems and updates have been introduced and have revolutionized management of T1DM. In early 2017, the Centers for Medicare & Medicaid Services (CMS) determined that CGM systems that are FDA approved for treatment decisions could be eligible for Medicare coverage [10]. Recently the American Diabetes Association has endorsed use of CGMs in children and adolescents with T1DM to help improve glucose control while minimizing risk of hypoglycemia [11].

A CGM consists of an electrode sensor placed subcutaneously, a transmitter, and a receiver. The sensor detects glucose levels by electrochemical detection of glucose [9]. This sensor measures the glucose levels in the interstitial fluid and is attached to a transmitter that sends the data to a receiver. The glycemic data and trends are displayed on the receiver or on the pump screen of part of an integrated system.

Various sensors that have been used include biosensors, which involve the use of natural oxygen cofactor, artificial redox mediators, direct electron transfer between glucose oxidase and the electrode, and direct electro-oxidation of glucose [12]. The most commonly used method in CGM technology today uses electrochemical sensors because of increased sensitivity and accuracy [13]. Typically, this will use glucose oxidase (GOx) to detect glucose levels. This particular enzyme electrochemical sensor reaction has gained widespread use because GOx remains stable at variable pH values and temperatures. GOx, with the aid of a cofactor, facilitates transfer of electrons and production of hydrogen peroxide. The electrochemical sensor detects the number of electron transfers and, therefore, the number of glucose molecules present. Oxygen is important for this reaction to occur in the subcutaneous tissue. In the setting of poor perfusion or hypoxia, sensors may not be able to accurately detect glucose levels without appropriate levels of oxygen present [13,14]. Fluorescence-based sensors have also been used and are discussed in further detail below.

Current recommendations for BG monitoring advise 6–10 BG readings daily to guide insulin management of T1DM patients [15]. CGM systems allow for readings every five minutes approximately throughout the day and night and, thus, provide information about accurate trends that previously were not accessible. Additionally, with some of the new systems, routine BG checks for mealtime insulin dosing may be replaced with CGM readings. At this point in time, there is a recommendation to check a finger-stick BG manually to confirm hypoglycemia or if clinically warranted; however, this may change in the future as sensor accuracy continues to improve.

Accuracy of systems is a critical aspect of CGM use and system calibrations have typically been required to ensure accuracy of readings. With typical home glucometer use, there is approximately a 20% margin of error for BG measurements [16]. Additionally, it is important to remember, that finger-stick BG values measure glucose from capillary blood while CGM sensors measure glucose from the interstitial fluid in the subcutaneous fat. These compartments do have slightly different glucose values especially during periods of rapid change in glycemia. This discrepancy in measurement values is known as 'lag time' in which the interstitial fluid glucose levels are lagging behind the blood values by a median of 6.8 min and up to almost 10 min in some cases [17,18]. The accuracy of systems is typically reported as a mean absolute relative difference (MARD) which is determined using data from clinical trials and calculated by using the difference in the CGM measurement and concurrent reference measurement of glucose used in the study [19]. Currently available CGM systems are discussed further in the sections below with system comparisons outlined in Table 1.

Table 1. An overview of currently available CGM systems.

	Abbott Freestyle Libre	Dexcom G6	Medtronic Guardian Sensor 3	Senseonics Eversense
FDA Approved Age	18 years and up	2 years and up	14 to 75 years	18 years and up
MARD	9.4% [20]	9% [21]	8.7% [22]	8.8% [23]
Duration of use	14 days	10 days	7 days	90 days
Calibration	not required	not required, but can if desired	2 required daily, recommend 3–4 daily	2 required daily
Display options	Scanner	Receiver, Smartphone, Tandem X2; May share to 5 devices	Medtronic insulin pump, Smartphone; May share to 5 devices	Smartphone; May share to 5 devices
Warm up time	1 h	2 h	2 h	24 h
Alarms	no	yes	yes	yes
Approved insertion sites/procedure	arm	abdomen (2 years and older); upper buttocks (2–17 years)	abdomen	implanted in office, upper arm

3.1. Standalone

3.1.1. Abbott Freestyle CGM Systems

Abbott's first CGM was the Freestyle Navigator and was initially FDA approved in 2008. This product was then subsequently pulled when Abbott's newer system the Freestyle Libre Flash

CGM, which did not require patient calibration with glucose entry, came out in 2014. Recently, the system has been updated and may be worn for 14 days prior to requiring a new sensor. The sensors are factory calibrated and require no calibration for the duration of the 14-day wear period [14]. There is a 1 h warm up period for the device to start generating data. The data are transferred to the reader when it is brought in proximity to the sensor. The reader then displays the current blood sugar with an arrow indicating the direction of the glucose trend and the readings over the last 8 h. The sensor is able to hold 8 h of data and data may be lost if the reader is not used in more than 8 h. The reader can hold data for up to 90 days and may be uploaded using device software or accessed via an approved smartphone device and the Freestyle LibreLink application. The Freestyle Libre has been approved for insertion in the arm [24]. While in the US, it is approved by the FDA in patients greater than 18 years old, it has been cleared for pediatric patients ages four years and up in Europe and Australia [25].

3.1.2. Dexcom CGM Systems

Dexcom is a company that focuses solely on CGM technology for diabetes patients. They first came out with their Short-Term Sensor (STS) system in 2006. In 2015, they released the Dexcom G4 Platinum CGM system. This system consists of a small sensor that measures glucose levels subcutaneously, a transmitter that is attached to the top of the sensor, and a receiver which displays the glucose readings and trends. With the introduction of their G4 system, Dexcom added share technology so that BG readings and trends may be monitored remotely via smartphone. The system originally worked exclusively with iOS systems, but is now compatible with some android devices. The Dexcom G5 system allowed users to bypass the receiver altogether and directly send data from the sensor/transmitter unit to their smartphone. The newest iteration, the Dexcom G6, can integrate with Tandem and display CGM data on the Tandem X2 insulin pump.

In March 2018, Dexcom released the G6 CGM system that is FDA approved for patients as young as two years old [26]. The G6 is factory calibrated with no need for calibration or finger-sticks to make clinical decisions based on FDA approval. Additionally, the G6 system is approved for wear up to 10 days. Through the smartphone application or receiver, alarms can be set for glucose target ranges to alert the user to episodes of hypoglycemia or hyperglycemia. Additionally, data may be shared with more than one smartphone device allowing parents and caregivers to remotely monitor the patient's glucose measurements.

3.1.3. Senseonics Eversense CGM System

Senseonics Eversense is the only implantable CGM device currently on the market. The device consists of an implantable sensor, removable transmitter, and a smartphone application. The transmitter activates the sensor which flashes an LED light source exciting the fluorescent polymer coating on the outside of the sensor. Glucose in the interstitial fluid will reversibly bind to the coating and alter the amount of light emitted by the polymer coating. The amount of emitted light is proportional to interstitial glucose concentration and is measured by photodetectors inside the sensor. The smart transmitter is attached to the skin with an adhesive, sitting directly over the sensor, and vibrates for alerts including hypoglycemia even when the smartphone is not in range. The transmitter is rechargeable and does not need to be replaced every three months with the implantable sensor. The implantation process can be done in the outpatient office setting by trained health care professionals. There is a 24-h warm up period after the sensor is initially placed followed by an initialization period that requires multiple calibrations within another 12-h period. Thereafter, the system requires two calibrations daily and advises finger-stick checks for treatment decisions regarding hypoglycemia or hyperglycemia. The transmitter does require charging daily that takes approximately 15 min to complete. The transmitter is water resistant up to a depth of 3.3 feet for 30 min at a time; however, the user needs to avoid submersion for the first five days of wear [27].

In the PRECISE study, Eversense was tested in 71 adults with type 1 and type 2 diabetes in multiple European countries. The mean absolute relative difference (MARD), a standard measure of

CGM accuracy, was 11.1% with a similar error profile to current CGM technology [28]. Following the initial study, the calibration methods were updated and a follow up study called PRECISE II was performed. This study was a multicenter US, nonrandomized, blinded trial in 90 adults and reported a MARD of 8.8% [23]. The in-development closed loop system iLet works in conjunction with the Eversense CGM system [29].

3.2. CGM Integrated with Insulin Pumps

Medtronic CGM Systems

As mentioned before, the Medtronic Minimed CGM was released in 1999 and was the first FDA-approved CGM device available. This system included a subcutaneous glucose sensor, a monitor, a connecting cable, and a ComStation compatible with Windows 95. It was updated to include alarms for hyperglycemia and hypoglycemia with a new device name, the Guardian Real-time CGM system. The next Medtronic system approved in 2016 was the Medtronic Minimed iPro2 system and was designed to be compatible with the Medtronic 530G insulin pump system.

The most recent Medtronic CGM system is the Guardian Sensor 3 system and works in conjunction with the Medtronic 670G insulin pump utilizing hybrid closed loop technology or with the Medtronic 630G insulin pump providing low glucose suspend. The Guardian Sensor 3 requires calibration at least twice daily, but recommends 3–4 calibrations per day for optimal accuracy. The new system does not require the purchase of a separate receiver, but directly transmits data via Bluetooth to the Medtronic insulin pump and/or an approved smartphone with the Medtronic application. The Medtronic Guardian Sensor 3 CGM can also be used in conjunction with insulin injections and features prediction of highs and lows with an alert 10–60 min prior to hyper- or hypoglycemia [30]. This sensor can alert patients to glucose changes via their smartphone or smartwatch similar to SMS messaging.

3.3. Limitations

Continuous glucose monitor systems have improved the monitoring of BGs for T1DM patients and allowed medical providers, caregivers, and patients access to BG trends that would otherwise be missed. However, there are significant limitations that must be considered with CGM systems. The cost of a CGM system can be prohibitive for patients who are uninsured or for whom insurance does not cover CGM. There are not only initial costs for the transmitter and receiver set up, but also monthly costs for sensor and transmitter replacement. Typically, sensors will last from 7–14 days depending on the CGM model. Transmitters additionally may need to be replaced monthly to a couple times per year. Since 2017, Medicaid has started to cover CGM costs with commercial insurance groups beginning to cover CGM prior to that time.

Continuous glucose monitors also require an additional body site for insertion away from an insulin pump site or injection site. In children and adults, CGM devices only have approval in particular sites. For the pediatric population, typically this is in the abdomen or gluteus. Patients however often need to interchange between multiple insertion sites most often in the abdomen, gluteus, or bilateral arms. There seems to be no difference in accuracy between sites among pediatric patients [31]. CGM systems over time have shown a variable degree of water resistance; therefore, patients need to pay attention to specific system capabilities: Abbott Freestyle Libre is water resistant to 3 feet for up to 30 min, Dexcom G6 sensor/transmitter are water resistant, Medtronic Guardian Sensor 3 is water resistant to 8 feet for up to 30 min, and Senseonics Eversense is water resistant to 3.3 feet for up to 30 min [25–27,30]. Due to the need for Bluetooth technology to transmit data to the receiver, CGMs may lose contact during water-based activities, such as showers, baths, and swimming [26]. During times when data is not being received, alerts based on glucose values will not be functional.

While glucose measurements are comparable during times of homeostasis between CGM systems and finger-stick glucose values, CGMs can lag behind when rapid glucose changes occur. Like all populations, patients with T1DM are encouraged to engage in physical activity for their overall health.

However, sudden changes in glucose might pose a challenge to current CGM capacity to accurately depict glucose trends and forewarn patients of impending hypoglycemia during or after physical activity. Zaharieva et al. reported a case study where they had a 40-year-old patient with T1DM who wore a Medtronic 670G pump and CGM integrated system, a Dexcom G5, and an Abbott Freestyle Libre during exercise. The patient performed one hour of moderate intensity running and monitored glucose values through the CGM systems and finger-stick measurements. All three of the CGM systems lagged behind finger-stick values when glucose values dropped during exercise with the largest difference in glucose levels noted in the first 30 min of exercise [32]. Additional studies have supported the finding that discrepancies between CGM and finger-stick values are greatest during exercise and return to previous accuracy within a couple hours after aerobic exercise [33].

3.4. Future Directions

Continuous glucose monitors have improved immensely in the last 20 years of clinical care. Future CGMs will need to improve upon the lag time of current devices to allow for better monitoring and management during physical exercise and periods of rapid glucose changes. As these products continue to develop, sensors and transmitters will likely become smaller and lower profile to skin for ease of wearability. Additionally, new adhesive strategies need to be employed to keep these devices in place as the lifetime of a sensor continues to improve. CGMs are already being used in hybrid closed-loop systems with insulin pumps; simultaneously, more collaborations are ongoing to make currently available CGM devices compatible with other independent insulin pumps with the goal of developing closed loop and suspend before low systems in the near future.

4. Insulin Pumps

Currently, it is estimated that more than one million people worldwide use an insulin pump for diabetes management including nearly 400,000 patients with T1DM in the US [34]. Insulin pumps are small devices that deliver short acting insulin subcutaneously via a small cannula self-placed by the patient every few days. They are designed to provide a near-continuous low dose of insulin delivered frequently in small boluses to mimic the actions of the β cells of the pancreas and also allow for bolus delivery of insulin at meal times or when needed for rapid correction of glucose. Insulin is given through a small tube called a cannula that is inserted into the subcutaneous tissue with a small needle and taped to the skin. Some insulin pump systems have tubing that runs from the device's insulin reservoir to the insertion site and some insulin pumps are tubing free. Tubing free systems stick directly to the skin with a cannula inserted into the subcutaneous tissue below the pump.

The pump itself is a battery-powered programmable device that holds multiple settings. Providers and patients are able to program multiple insulin delivery settings based on the time of day and in multiple profiles. Within a profile, there will be basal rates for 24-h, and typically a programmed carb ratio and insulin sensitivity factor with a target glucose. Additionally, settings may include insulin action time to allow the pump to calculate current insulin activity when giving additional boluses. Most pumps contain an insulin reservoir that typically is in a cylindrical shape. When the user programs the pump to deliver insulin, the plunger is pushed by the pump's internal mechanisms to precisely deliver the amount of insulin desired. The Tandem insulin pumps, however, use a bag reservoir for the insulin to allow for a smaller pump size.

The first insulin pump was designed by Dr. Arnold Kadish in the 1960s and was the size of a large backpack. In the 1970s, Dean Kamen introduced the AS2C, also known as the 'blue brick', and later the 'autosyringe.' These initial systems were large and often difficult to use even requiring a screwdriver to adjust insulin doses. By the mid-1980s, smaller and more precise systems were starting to emerge [35]. A large producer of insulin pumps, Animas announced in 2017 that it would be discontinuing insulin pump production and support. The insulin pump market has continued to evolve and now has three major companies producing insulin pumps in the US: Medtronic, Insulet, and Tandem. There are multiple other insulin pump brands out on the market and in development worldwide, including Cellnovo, Kaleido, Roche Diagnostics Accu-Chek, and Sooil Dana Diabecare systems discussed below.

A major advantage of insulin pumps is that they allow patients to avoid multiple daily injections. Some pumps have even featured remote bolus programming allowing for parents of pediatric patients a convenient way to dose insulin for active kids. Additionally, insulin pumps allow for variable basal rates throughout the day. Circadian rhythms affect insulin requirements over a 24-h period and these differences can be more pronounced in pubertal patients [36]. Pumps certainly allow for better accommodation of differences in circadian rhythm than is possible with a long acting insulin administered once to twice daily. Insulin pumps allow for precise delivery of small insulin doses with some pumps even allowing for dosing changes down to increments of 0.01 units and minimal insulin delivery of 0.025 units per hour which may be helpful in very young patients who are often very sensitive to insulin. Furthermore, some providers have argued that use of U10 (1/10th the concentration) insulin instead of standard U100 insulin in insulin pumps could improve precision by allowing delivery of very small doses [37]. However, others argue that insulin delivery is not truly continuous, but is delivered frequently in small boluses to mimic endogenous basal production. Therefore, the option for diluted insulin or very small basal dose increments may not change care in clinical practice.

When considering insulin pump therapy, accuracy of insulin delivery is also an important consideration. Insulin pump manufacturers specify delivery accuracy to ±5% of insulin dose entered by using an international standard method. Typically these evaluations look at an average of the accuracy over 100 consecutive boluses within the system of interest. A 2013 study looked at insulin delivery accuracy of three conventional insulin pumps and one patch insulin pump by testing bolus accuracy in these systems. They noted a statistically significant difference in accuracy between the traditional systems and patch insulin pump with better single-dose accuracy noted in the traditional insulin pumps [38]. A standard measure of insulin pump accuracy, IEC 60601-2-24, helps to provide consistent testing of systems, but some researchers argue that this measure may be incomplete and alternative measures are being proposed [39].

Most importantly, pumps have been shown to improve glycemic control resulting in a lower HbA1c. In a recent study of pediatric patients with T1DM, patients with insulin pump therapy were shown to have lower rates of severe hypoglycemia, lower incidence of diabetic ketoacidosis, lower HbA1c, and lower total daily insulin doses than matched patients on multiple daily insulin injection therapy [40]. Insulin pumps allow patients increased flexibility in their routines and account of insulin action time thereby reducing the risk of insulin stacking. Temporary basal rates can be used to decrease hourly insulin during or after intense exercise. Patients are able to give multiple doses without requiring additional injections and utilize variable bolus settings for high fat meals. In the following sections, currently available insulin pumps are introduced and Table 2 provides a comparison of systems available within the US.

Table 2. An overview of currently available insulin pump systems within the US.

	Medtronic 670G	OmniPod DASH	Tandem X2
Ages approved	7 years and above	All ages	6 years and above
Dosing increments	Basal: 0.025 units/hour; Bolus: 0.025 units	Basal: 0.05 units/hour; Bolus: 0.5 units	Basal: 0.001 units/hour at greater than 0.1 units/hour; Bolus: 0.01 units at greater than 0.05 units
Tubing	Tubing lengths—18″, 23″, and 32″ Can be disconnected from infusion site	Patch, Tubeless	Tubing lengths—23″, 32″, and 43″ Can be disconnected from infusion site
CGM integration	Medtronic Guardian Sensor 3	Dexcom G5/G6	Dexcom G5/G6
Hypoglycemia prevention	Yes, low glucose suspend with Sensor 3	No	Yes, Basal-IQ with G6 only
Closed Loop Available	Yes, Auto-mode	No	No

4.1. Medtronic Insulin Pumps

Medtronic was founded initially in 1949 as a medical device repair shop. In 1983, they released their first insulin pump to the market, the Minimed 502. Over the next several years, they launched updates to insertion sites and infusion sets that allowed for temporary detachment from the pump system. In 2003, they introduced the BolusWizard which wirelessly shared the glucose value from the system-integrated glucometer and suggested an insulin dose. In 2006, they released the MiniMed Paradigm Real-Time System that integrated CGM data for viewing on the insulin pump display. In 2013, the FDA approved the MiniMed 530G with Enlite for patients greater than age 16 years. This was the first system available in the US that provided 'Threshold Suspend' automation and would stop insulin delivery for up to two hours if the glucose level reached a preset low limit with no user response to the alert. The 630G was released in 2016 and was followed quickly by their most recent insulin pump the Medtronic 670G System [41].

The Medtronic 670G system features two operational modes: manual mode in which the system acts as a traditional pump, and auto mode in which the system acts as a hybrid closed loop device using CGM input to alter basal insulin output. The Medtronic 670G system will be discussed in greater detail below.

4.2. OmniPod Insulin Pumps

Insulet Corporation, the maker of OmniPod, was founded in 2000 and first received FDA clearance for OmniPod in 2005. This system was the first developed 'patch' insulin pump with two components: a disposable OmniPod infusion pump and the OmniPod Personal Diabetes Manager (PDM) [42]. The PDM is a handheld battery-powered device that controls insulin delivery from the disposable infusion pump. The infusion pump can be worn for up to 3 days and is waterproof up to 25 feet for 60 min. It will deliver insulin based on the programmed basal rates set up in the PDM. The PDM communicates wirelessly with the infusion pump and needs to be within five feet to give a bolus insulin delivery or change previously set basal insulin delivery rates.

The most recent iteration, OmniPod DASH, is anticipated for wide availability in early 2019 [43]. This system uses Bluetooth technology for communication between the PDM and infusion pump and allows users to view their PDM data on mobile phone applications. Additionally, with the smartphone applications, users will be able to share data with up to 12 people. The application will integrate Dexcom G6 CGM data with insulin delivery data on a single screen for streamlined analysis of information. However, the user will still need the PDM to make basal rate delivery changes or to give bolus insulin doses.

4.3. Tandem Insulin Pumps

In 2008, Tandem Diabetes Care, Inc. was founded from a previous company Phluid, Inc. [44]. The t:slim insulin pump received FDA clearance in 2011 and was the first ever touchscreen insulin pump. In 2015, they received FDA approval for integration with the Dexcom G4 CGM system. The t:slim, via Bluetooth technology, offered Dexcom G4 CGM data display on the insulin pump screen. This allowed for data to be interpreted in real-time with only one device. The newest Tandem product, the X2, was released in 2016.

The Tandem X2 insulin pump features integration with Dexcom G5 or G6 CGM systems. They use Basal-IQ technology to reduce incidence of hypoglycemia in patients using both the X2 insulin pump and a Dexcom G6 CGM. The PROLOG trial showed significantly reduced rates of hypoglycemia without rebound hyperglycemia with use of the Tandem Basal-IQ system. The algorithm works by predicting glucose levels 30 min into the future and suspends insulin delivery if the predicted glucose value is <80 mg/dL or the actual glucose value is <70 mg/dL [45]. Updates of the Tandem insulin pump will be through software updates that can be downloaded to the patient's pump as new systems are released.

4.4. Insulin Pumps Systems Available Only Outside of the US

4.4.1. Cellnovo Insulin Pumps

The Cellnovo system is an insulin pump available to patients in Europe, but not currently available in the US. The system is comprised of a small insulin pump that is controlled via Bluetooth technology with a locked down Android device. The pump has short tubing and uses an adhesive to attach to the skin. It is water resistant to a depth of 36 feet for up to 1 h. This system also includes an activity tracker and food library, as well as applications for data management [46].

4.4.2. Kaleido Insulin Pumps

The Kaleido insulin pump is newly available in Europe at this point. Some of this pump's unique features include the option of placing the infusion site with variable lengths of tubing to accommodate for different locations on the body and the insulin pump can be placed on the skin with an adhesive or placed in a pocket. Also, the system comes with two rechargeable pumps that can be used interchangeably and a handset that controls insulin delivery via Bluetooth technology. The pumps are water resistant up to a depth of 3.3 feet for up to 1 h; however, the pump charging station and handset must be kept dry. Kaleido also offers 10 color options for the insulin pump [47].

4.4.3. Roche Diagnostics Accu-Chek Insulin Pumps

The Accu-Chek Combo system first became available in the US in 2012 following approval by the FDA. The system was comprised of an insulin pump and glucometer that was connected via Bluetooth technology. The Accu-Chek insulin pumps are no longer supported in the US; however, they are still prominent in Europe and continue to support glucometers within the US. Their most recent systems, the Accu-Chek Spirit Combo and Accu-Chek Insight, are currently supported in many countries around the world and offer some advantages. The systems, comprised of an insulin pump and smart glucometer, allow the patient to change pump settings and use a bolus calculator without directly changing settings on the pump by input through the Bluetooth connected glucometer. The Accu-Chek Insight also allows patients to use pre-filled insulin cartridges instead of filling cartridges manually when replacing insulin [48].

4.4.4. Sooil Dana Diabecare Insulin Pumps

The Sooil Company has two insulin pumps currently on the market, Dana Diabecare R and Dana Diabecare RS insulin pumps. They are currently available in multiple countries in Europe and Asia. The Dana Diabecare R model features a connected glucometer and lightweight design. The system also allows for remote control of pump settings through an Android based smartphone application [49]. The Dana Diabecare RS system was released in 2018 and connects with smartphone applications for both Android and iOS systems via Bluetooth technology [50].

4.5. Limitations

Insulin pumps have revolutionized insulin delivery by allowing for very precise insulin dosing and small dose delivery, but there are limitations to therapy. Cost is an important issue in care of patients with T1DM. In the DIAMOND study, researchers enrolled 75 adults with T1DM already using CGM and randomized them to either insulin pump therapy or continued multiple daily injections (MDI) therapy and followed these patients for 28 weeks [51]. They reported total per person costs for the length of the trial as $8272 for patients in the CGM + insulin pump group and $5623 for patients in the CGM + MDI group. Insulin pump therapy is often covered by insurance with improvement of out of pocket costs, but has associated monthly costs for supplies required for pump therapy including infusion sets, tubing, adhesives, batteries, insulin reservoirs or cartridges, and insulin.

At this point, many insulin pumps are considered 'open-loop', meaning that the device acts based on settings that have been programmed into the system and cannot alter its output based on the effect of insulin on glucose. This requires careful monitoring of glucose values during therapy and a well-trained patient or parent who can alter insulin pump settings to vary insulin delivery based on clinical need.

With insulin pump therapy, there has always been a concern for increased risk of diabetic ketoacidosis (DKA), a life-threatening complication of T1DM. Since insulin pumps utilize short-acting insulin, with pump site failure or disconnection, patients would not have the safety of subcutaneously injected long acting insulin to prevent DKA. In 2007, a consensus statement from the European Society for Paediatric Endocrinology issued a warning that 'individuals using continuous subcutaneous insulin infusion (CSII) are potentially at increased risk of developing DKA, with DKA rates varying from 2.7–9 episodes per 100 patient-years' [52]. More recently, Dogan et al. shared data from 205 adult T1DM patients treated with insulin pump therapy from 2006 to 2015. They noted only 10 cases of DKA in nine of their patients throughout the course of the study which indicates an incidence of 1.0 case/100 patient years which is reassuring [53]. Additionally, Hoshina et al. noted similar risk of DKA between patients using insulin pump versus multiple daily injection methods. Interestingly, they reported significantly lower rates of DKA in insulin pump patients who received care at a practice with experience caring for more than 250 insulin pump patients [54].

4.6. Future Directions

Over the last 50 years, insulin pumps have continued to advance and improve now with more precision and convenience than ever before. As these systems continue to evolve, more closed-loop systems will emerge onto the market. Multiple closed-loop systems are currently in development with unique algorithms designed to deliver insulin based on glucose levels measured with a connected CGM system.

Bihormonal therapy with glucagon and insulin working together has long been discussed as ideal to mimic the endogenous functioning pancreas. The iLet Bionic Pancreas which plans to utilize both glucagon and insulin has been in development for several years [55]. In a randomized controlled trial, bihormonal pump therapy was compared with insulin only pump therapy showing improvement in mean blood glucose and reduction in incidence of hypoglycemia [56].

5. Hybrid Closed-Loop Insulin Delivery Systems

With the emergence of the first commercially available hybrid closed-loop system, the Medtronic 670G, diabetes care advanced a step closer to development of an artificial pancreas. These systems have been shown to increase the percentage of time in glucose range for users. In a 2010 study, OmniPod and Freestyle Navigator CGM were used to compare an open- versus closed-loop system showing an improvement from 64% to 78% time within range for users [57]. Additionally, multiple studies have shown reduction in incidence and severity of hypoglycemia in patients using closed-loop systems in both pediatric and adult patients [58,59]. Multiple algorithms are under development for use in hybrid closed-loop systems. Release of new hybrid closed-loop systems including the OmniPod Horizon, the Tandem Control-IQ, and the Beta Bionics iLet, is anticipated in the next couple of years.

There are currently four main types of control algorithms being employed in the development of closed loop systems. Model predictive control (MPC) algorithms are the most commonly used and aim to predict glucose levels in the near future and adjust insulin delivery based on that prediction. Another algorithm is the proportional integral derivative type which responds to real-time measured glucose values. Fuzzy logic algorithms determine insulin doses based on CGM data in the way that an expert clinician would make insulin adjustments. There are also bio-inspired algorithms that utilize a mathematical model to determine insulin doses based on how β cells would act in response to glucose in the body [60].

5.1. Currently Available

Medtronic

The Medtronic 670G is the only hybrid closed-loop system currently available on the market and is approved in the US and Europe in patients 7 years and up. This hybrid system uses the Guardian 3 sensor as well as SmartGuard technology during Auto mode to adjust insulin basal rates to help keep glucose levels within target range. Basal insulin delivery is adjusted every five minutes based on CGM readings to increase time within range. Additionally, the suspend before low feature, that can also be used in manual mode, stops insulin up to 30 min prior to reaching a preset low glucose value. The insulin delivery will automatically restart when glucose levels have recovered to avoid rebound hyperglycemia.

The system requires patients to enter carbohydrate corrections at meal-times similar to a traditional pump when in Auto Mode. For CGM operation and use in Auto Mode, patients must calibrate with finger-stick glucose values every 12 h and when alerted by the pump to do so. However, at this time, the system does not allow for sharing of real time CGM data with friends or family. In their pivotal trial, they reported a decrease in average Hb A1c values from 7.4% to 6.9% and an increase in time within desired glucose range (70 mg/dL to 180 mg/dL) from 66.7% to 72.2% of the time [61]. Stone et al. provide a further review of the Medtronic 670G Hybrid Closed-Loop System [62].

5.2. Anticipated in the Next 1–2 Years

5.2.1. Beta Bionics

Beta Bionics is currently working on the iLet system that would allow for infusion of both insulin and glucagon in response to CGM data. The company is working with Senseonics Eversense CGM which is a physician subcutaneously implanted device that would read glucose levels for up to 3 months [29]. Initial release of the system is anticipated in 2020 as an insulin-only device with addition of glucagon anticipated in the next couple of years. In their 2017 study, they noted glycemic differences in the bihormonal treatment group versus traditional pump therapy including average CGM glucose of 140 mg/dL vs. 162 mg/dL and only 0.6% vs. 1.9% of time spent with glucose less than 60 mg/dL. They did, however, note an increase in complaints of nausea based on their scale scoring system [56].

5.2.2. OmniPod

The OmniPod Horizon Automated Glucose Control System is under development. The system uses Dexcom G6 CGM input and Insulet personal MPC algorithm. They presented the results of their clinic trial at the 2018 American Diabetes Association meeting, showing increased time in range and decreased hypoglycemia during both day and night in adults, adolescents, and children. Their initial study showed mean time less than 70 mg/dL 0.7% in adults and 2% in pediatric patients and percentage of time in the target range 69.5–73% in adult and pediatric age groups [63]. The system release is anticipated in 2019.

5.2.3. Tandem

In 2016, Tandem announced the plan for development of a closed-loop insulin delivery system called Control-IQ using Tandem X2 insulin pumps, Dexcom G6 CGM system, and TypeZero artificial pancreas (AP) technology [64]. Their initial pilot study published in December 2018 included five adult patients with well-controlled T1DM and showed mean time in range of 86% overall, mean glucose of 130 mg/dL, and median time less than 70 mg/dL of 2.8% [65]. They have recently completed another clinical trial of the Control-IQ system and will likely submit results for FDA approval in the coming months. The new system is anticipated later in 2019.

5.3. Limitations

The current technology allows for closed-loop insulin delivery response to glucose values and trends. However, at this point, users still need to check glucose values at least twice daily to calibrate the CGM device used in conjunction with the closed-loop system. Additionally, currently available systems require users to manually give bolus insulin for meal times by entering in carbohydrates and the current glucose value from either CGM or finger-stick value.

For the currently available system the Medtronic 670G, options for glucose goals are limited while in Auto Mode to 120 mg/dL or 150 mg/dL. For many pediatric patients who experience hypoglycemia following exercise, an elevated glucose target of 150 mg/dL may be insufficient to prevent hypoglycemia. Conversely, for older patients who can achieve very tight glycemic control, a target of 120 mg/dL may be higher than desired. Patients have adapted to the system by giving 'fake' carbohydrate boluses to achieve tighter control; however, this practice could lead to increased risk of hypoglycemia in the user [66].

5.4. Future Directions

Hybrid closed-loop systems are still new to the market with multiple new systems anticipated in the coming years. Across the globe, several systems are currently in development or undergoing clinical trials and may be several years away from introduction into the market. Previous reviews have detailed systems in development extensively including the papers from Trevitt et al. and Bekiari et al. and should be referenced for a more detailed overview of anticipated systems [60,67]. As this technology continues to develop further, systems will ideally require less and less management from the patient and the provider. As systems move forward, length of time they may be worn will likely increase. Additionally, integrated CGM systems will require less calibration and significantly less finger-sticks.

As these systems continue to progress, meal-time insulin may no longer be required and therefore the patient would not be required to enter carbohydrates consumed. Studies have started to look at unannounced meals in the setting of hybrid closed-loop insulin delivery systems. In a study done by Cameron et al., patients wore a closed-loop system in a hospital setting and a hotel setting and challenged the system with unannounced meals and exercise. During the study, they were able to report daytime mean glucose of 158 mg/dL showing promising results for a future system [68]. Forlenza et al. further investigated with both adults and adolescents in a hotel setting. In their study, they tested an Android-based AP system with six adults and 4 adolescents in the setting of exercise and unannounced meals. Although they showed overall mean CGM data of 157 mg/dL throughout the study, they did note a significantly lower CGM value following announced versus unannounced meals at 140 mg/dL versus 197 mg/dL. Meal announcement is still superior in glycemic control at this time given current insulin pharmacokinetics, CGM accuracy and lag, and possible speed of insulin delivery in current systems [69].

In recent studies, bihormonal pump therapy has shown improvement in mean blood glucose and reduction in incidence of hypoglycemia in comparison with insulin only pump therapy [56]. In the pursuit of bihormonal pump development, glucagon still is unstable in extended time periods in liquid form. In the future, we will likely see the emergence of a bihormonal closed-loop system using both insulin and glucagon, possibly as a standard of care.

6. Conclusions

Type 1 Diabetes is a chronic disease requiring glucose monitoring and intensive insulin therapy. Diabetes technology has continually evolved over the years to improve quality of life and ease of care for affected patients. Continuous glucose monitors allow patients to observe and discern trends in their glycemic control. These devices also give peace of mind with preset alerts for hypoglycemia and the ability for family or friends to follow a patient's glucose trends. The major products available and in use today are the Abbott Freestyle Libre, the Dexcom G6, the Medtronic Guardian Sensor 3, and the Senseonics Eversense.

Insulin pumps have continued to improve and innovate since their emergence into the market. Pumps allow patients to infuse insulin for up to 3 days without giving individual insulin injections. These devices allow for very low doses in pediatric patients and varied basal rates during different times of day and during different activities. They also allow for more freedom in dietary schedule and multiple carbohydrate-based doses in addition to mealtimes. Hybrid closed-loop systems have harnessed the data gathered with CGM use to aid in basal insulin dosing and hypoglycemia prevention. As technology continues to progress, patients will likely have to enter less and less information into their pump systems manually.

In the future, we will likely see a system that requires no manual patient input and allows users to eat throughout the day without counting carbohydrates or entering in any blood sugars. As technology continues to advance, endocrinologists and diabetes providers need to stay current to better guide their patients in optimal use of emerging management tools.

Funding: The authors received no funding for this manuscript.

Conflicts of Interest: The authors declare no conflict of interest.

References

1. The DCCT/EDIC Research Group. Intensive diabetes treatment and cardiovascular outcomes in type 1 diabetes: The DCCT/EDIC Study 30-year follow-up. *Diabetes Care* **2016**, *39*, 686–693. [CrossRef] [PubMed]
2. Lakhtakia, R. The history of diabetes mellitus. *Sultan Qaboos Univ. Med. J.* **2013**, *13*, 368–370. [CrossRef] [PubMed]
3. Quianzon, C.C.; Cheikh, I. History of insulin. *J. Community Hosp. Intern. Med. Perspect.* **2012**, *2*. [CrossRef] [PubMed]
4. van Beers, C.A.; DeVries, J.H.; Kleijer, S.J.; Smits, M.M.; Geelhoed-Duijvestijn, P.H.; Kramer, M.H.; Diamant, M.; Snoek, F.J.; Serne, E.H. Continuous glucose monitoring for patients with type 1 diabetes and impaired awareness of hypoglycaemia (IN CONTROL): A randomised, open-label, crossover trial. *Lancet Diabetes Endocrinol.* **2016**, *4*, 893–902. [CrossRef]
5. van Beers, C.A.; DeVries, J.H. Continuous Glucose Monitoring: Impact on Hypoglycemia. *J. Diabetes Sci. Technol.* **2016**, *10*, 1251–1258. [CrossRef] [PubMed]
6. Heinemann, L.; Freckmann, G.; Ehrmann, D.; Faber-Heinemann, G.; Guerra, S.; Waldernmaier, D.; Hermanns, N. Real-time continuous glucose monitoring in adults with type 1 diabetes and impaired hypoglycaemia awareness or severe hypoglycaemia treated with multiple daily insulin injections (HypoDE): A multicentre, randomised, controlled trial. *Lancet* **2018**, *391*, 1367–1377. [CrossRef]
7. Burckhardt, M.A.; Roberts, A.; Smith, G.J.; Abraham, M.B.; Davis, E.A.; Jones, T.W. The Use of Continuous Glucose Monitoring with Remote Monitoring Improves Psychosocial Measures in Parents of Children with Type 1 Diabetes: A Randomized Crossover Trial. *Diabetes Care* **2018**, *41*, 2641–2643. [CrossRef]
8. Olczuk, D.; Priefer, R. A history of continuous glucose monitors (CGMs) in self-monitoring of diabetes mellitus. *Diabetes Metab. Syndr.* **2018**, *12*, 181–187. [CrossRef] [PubMed]
9. Liebl, A.; Henrichs, H.R.; Heinemann, L.; Freckmann, G.; Biermann, E.; Thomas, A. Continuous Glucose Monitoring Group of the Working Group Diabetes Technology of the German Diabetes Association. Continuous glucose monitoring: Evidence and consensus statement for clinical use. *J. Diabetes Sci. Technol.* **2013**, *7*, 500–519. [CrossRef]
10. Tucker, M. Diabetes Forecast. Available online: http://www.diabetesforecast.org/2018/02-mar-apr/medicare-coverage-for.html (accessed on 12 January 2019).
11. American Diabetes Association. Standards of Medical Care in Diabetes. Chapter 13 Children and Adolescents. *Diabetes Care* **2019**, *42* (Suppl. 1), S148–S164. [CrossRef]
12. Vaddiraju, S.; Burgess, D.J.; Tomazos, I.; Jain, F.C.; Papadimitrakopoulos, F. Technologies for Continuous Glucose Monitoring: Current Problems and Future Promises. *J. Diabetes Sci. Technol.* **2010**, *4*, 1540–1562. [CrossRef]

13. Yoo, E.H.; Lee, S.Y. Glucose biosensors: An overview of use in clinical practice. *Sensors* **2010**, *10*, 4558–4578. [CrossRef]

14. Bolinder, J.; Antuna, R.; Geelhoed-Duijvestijn, P.; Kroger, J.; Weitgasser, R. Novel glucose-sensing technology and hypoglycaemia in type 1 diabetes: A multicenter, non-masked, randomised controlled trial. *Lancet* **2016**, *388*, 2254–2263. [CrossRef]

15. Chiang, J.L.; Maahs, D.M.; Garvey, K.C.; Hood, K.K.; Laffel, L.M.; Weinzimer, S.A.; Wolfsdorf, J.I.; Schatz, D. Type 1 Diabetes in Children and Adolescents: A Position Statement by the American Diabetes Association. *Diabetes Care* **2018**, *41*, 2026–2044. [CrossRef]

16. Freckmann, G.; Schmid, C.; Baumstark, A.; Pleus, S.; Link, M.; Haug, C. System accuracy evaluation of 43 blood glucose monitoring systems for self-monitoring of blood glucose according to DIN EN ISO 15197. *J. Diabetes Sci. Technol.* **2012**, *6*, 1060–1075. [CrossRef]

17. Basu, A.; Dube, S.; Slama, M.; Errazuriz, I.; Amezcua, J.C.; Kudva, T.C.; Peyser, T.; Carter, R.E.; Cobelli, C.; Basu, R. Time Lag of Glucose from Intravascular to Interstitial Compartment in Humans. *Diabetes* **2013**, *62*, 4083–4087. [CrossRef]

18. Basu, A.; Dube, S.; Veettil, S.; Slama, M.; Kudva, Y.; Peyser, T.; Carter, R.; Cobelli, C.; Basu, R. Time lag of glucose from intravascular to interstitial compartment in type 1 diabetes. *J. Diabetes Sci. Technol.* **2015**, *9*, 63–68. [CrossRef]

19. Reiterer, F.; Polterauer, P.; Schoemaker, M.; Schmelzeisen-Redecker, G.; Freckmann, G.; Heinemann, L.; del Re, L. Significance and reliability of MARD for the accuracy of CGM systems. *J. Diabetes Sci. Technol.* **2017**, *11*, 59–67. [CrossRef]

20. Abbott Diabetes Care. Available online: https://provider.myfreestyle.com/freestyle-libre-clinical-evidence.html (accessed on 4 March 2019).

21. Shah, V.N.; Laffel, L.M.; Wadwa, R.P.; Garg, S.K. Performance of a factory-calibrated real-time continuous glucose monitoring system utilizing an automated sensor applicator. *Diabetes Technol. Ther.* **2018**, *20*, 428–433. [CrossRef]

22. Medtronic Diabetes. Available online: https://professional.medtronicdiabetes.com/guardian-sensor-3 (accessed on 4 March 2019).

23. Christiansen, M.P.; Klaff, L.J.; Brazg, R.; Chang, A.R.; Levy, C.J.; Lam, D.; Denham, D.S.; Atlee, G.; Bode, B.W.; Walters, S.J.; et al. A Prospective Multicenter Evaluation of the Accuracy of a Novel Implanted Continuous Glucose Sensor: PRECISE II. *Diabetes Technol. Ther.* **2018**, *20*, 197–206. [CrossRef] [PubMed]

24. Brown, A.; Close, K. Diatribe. Available online: https://diatribe.org/abbotts-freestyle-libre-approved-us-replace-routine-fingersticks (accessed on 13 January 2019).

25. Freestyle Libre. Available online: http://www.freestylelibrepro.us/patients.html (accessed on 13 January 2019).

26. Dexcom. Available online: https://www.dexcom.com/g6-cgm-system (accessed on 13 January 2019).

27. Senseonics. Available online: https://www.eversensediabetes.com/products/ (accessed on 3 March 2019).

28. Kropff, J.; Choudhary, P.; Neupane, S.; Barnard, K.; Bain, S.C.; Kapitza, C.; Forst, T.; Link, M.; Dehennis, A.; DeVries, J.H. Accuracy and Longevity of an Implantable Continuous Glucose Sensor in the PRECISE Study: A 180-Day, Prospective, Multicenter, Pivotal Trial. *Diabetes Care* **2017**, *40*, 63–68. [CrossRef]

29. Business Wire. Available online: https://www.businesswire.com/news/home/20180607005609/en/Senseonics-Beta-Bionics-Partner-Development-Bionic-Pancreas (accessed on 26 January 2019).

30. Medtronic Diabetes. Available online: https://www.medtronicdiabetes.com/products/guardian-connect-continuous-glucose-monitoring-system (accessed on 22 January 2019).

31. Faccioli, S.; Del Favero, S.; Visentin, R.; Bonfanti, R.; Iafusco, D.; Rabbone, I.; Marigliano, M.; Schiaffini, R.; Bruttomesso, D.; Cobelli, C.; et al. Accuracy of CGM Sensor in Pediatric Subjects with Type 1 Diabetes. Comparison of Three Insertion Sites: Arms, Abdomen, and Gluteus. *J. Diabetes Sci. Technol.* **2017**, *11*, 1147–1154. [CrossRef]

32. Zaharieva, D.P.; Riddell, M.C.; Henske, J. The Accuracy of Continuous Glucose Monitoring and Flash Glucose Monitoring During Aerobic Exercise in Type 1 Diabetes. *J. Diabetes Sci. Technol.* **2019**, *13*, 140–141. [CrossRef] [PubMed]

33. Biagi, L.; Bertachi, A.; Quiros, C.; Gimenez, M.; Conget, I.; Bondia, J.; Vehi, J. Accuracy of Continuous Glucose Monitoring before, during, and after Aerobic and Anaerobic Exercise in Patients with Type 1 Diabetes Mellitus. *Biosensors* **2018**, *8*, 22. [CrossRef] [PubMed]

34. American Diabetes Association. Available online: http://www.diabetes.org/newsroom/press-releases/2015/insulin-pumps.html (accessed on 20 January 2019).

35. Sherr, J.; Tamborlane, W.V. Past, Present, and Future of Insulin Pump Therapy: A Better Shot at Diabetes Control. *Mt. Sinai J. Med.* **2008**, *75*, 352–361. [CrossRef]

36. Bachran, R.; Beyer, P.; Klinkert, C.; Heidtmann, B.; Rosenbauer, J.; Holl, R.W.; German/Austrian DPV Initiative; German Pediatric CSII Working Group; BMBF Competence Network Diabetes. Basal rates and circadian profiles in continuous subcutaneous insulin infusion (CSII) differ for preschool children, prepubertal children, adolescents, and young adults. *Pediatr. Diabetes* **2012**, *13*, 1–5. [CrossRef] [PubMed]

37. Frohnert, B.I.; Alonso, G.T. Challenges in Delivering Smaller Doses of Insulin. *Diabetes Technol. Ther.* **2015**, *17*, 597–599. [CrossRef]

38. Jahn, L.G.; Capurro, J.J.; Levy, B.L. Comparative dose accuracy of durable and patch insulin infusion pumps. *J. Diabetes Sci. Technol.* **2013**, *7*, 1011–1020. [CrossRef] [PubMed]

39. Pleus, S.; Kamecke, U.; Waldenmaier, D.; Freckmann, G. Reporting insulin pump accuracy: Trumpet curves according to IEC 60601-2-24 and beyond. *J. Diabetes Sci. Technol.* **2018**. [CrossRef]

40. Karges, B.; Rosenbauer, J.; Holterhus, P.M.; Beyer, P.; Seithe, H.; Vogel, C.; Bockmann, A.; Peters, D.; Muther, S.; Neu, A.; et al. Hospital admission for diabetic ketoacidosis or severe hypoglycemia in 31,330 young patients with type 1 diabetes. *Eur. J. Endocrinol.* **2015**, *173*, 341–350. [CrossRef]

41. Medtronic. Available online: https://www.medtronic.com/us-en/about/history.html (accessed on 4 February 2019).

42. Zisser, H.C. The OmniPod Insulin Management System: The latest innovation in insulin pump therapy. *Diabetes Ther.* **2010**, *1*, 10–24. [CrossRef] [PubMed]

43. OmniPod. Available online: https://www.myomnipod.com/home (accessed on 26 January 2019).

44. San Diego Tribune. Available online: https://www.sandiegouniontribune.com/business/biotech/sdut-san-diegos-tandem-diabetics-sell-compact-insulin-p-2011nov16-story.html (accessed on 26 January 2019).

45. Forlenza, G.P.; Li, Z.; Buckingham, B.A.; Pinsker, J.E.; Cengiz, E.; Wadwa, R.P.; Ekhlaspour, L.; Church, M.M.; Weinzimer, S.A.; Jost, E.; et al. Predictive Low-Glucose Suspend Reduces Hypoglycemia in Adults, Adolescents, and Children with Type 1 Diabetes in an At-Home Randomized Crossover Study: Results of the PROLOG Trial. *Diabetes Care* **2018**, *41*, 2155–2161. [CrossRef] [PubMed]

46. Cellnovo. Available online: https://www.cellnovo.com/pump (accessed on 5 March 2019).

47. Kaleido. Available online: https://www.hellokaleido.com/en/about-kaleido (accessed on 5 March 2019).

48. Roche Diagnostics. Available online: https://www.accu-chek.co.uk/insulin-pumps/ (accessed on 5 March 2019).

49. Advanced Therapeutics. Available online: https://advancedtherapeutics.org.uk/shop/dana-diabecare-insulin-pump/238/ (accessed on 5 March 2019).

50. Advanced Therapeutics. Available online: https://advancedtherapeutics.org.uk/shop/dana-diabecare-insulin-pump/dana-rs-insulin-pump-2018 (accessed on 5 March 2019).

51. Wan, W.; Skandari, M.R.; Minc, A.; Nathan, A.G.; Winn, A.; Zarei, P.; O'Grady, M.; Huang, E.S. Cost-effectiveness of Continous Glucose Monitoring for Adults with Type 1 Diabetes Compared with Self-Monitoring of Blood Glucose: The DIAMOND Randomized Trial. *Diabetes Care* **2018**, *41*, 1227–1234. [CrossRef] [PubMed]

52. Phillip, M.; Battelino, T.; Rodriguez, H.; Danne, T.; Kaufman, F. Use of Insulin Pump Therapy in the Pediatric Age-Group. *Diabetes Care* **2007**, *30*, 1653–1662. [CrossRef] [PubMed]

53. Dogan, A.D.A.; Jorgensen, U.L.; Gjessing, H.J. Diabetic Ketoacidosis Among Patients Treated with Continuous Subcutaneous Insulin Infusion. *J. Diabetes Sci. Technol.* **2017**, *11*, 631–632. [CrossRef] [PubMed]

54. Hoshina, S.; Andersen, G.S.; Jorgensen, M.E.; Ridderstrale, M.; Vistisen, D.; Andersen, H.U. Treatment modality-dependent risk of diabetic ketoacidosis in patients with type 1 diabetes: Danish adult database study. *Diabetes Technol. Ther.* **2018**, *20*, 229–234. [CrossRef]

55. Brown, A.; Wolf, A.; Close, K. Diatribe. Available online: https://diatribe.org/introducing-beta-bionics-bringing-ilet-bionic-pancreas-market (accessed on 26 January 2019).

56. El-Khatib, F.H.; Balliro, C.; Hillard, M.A.; Magyar, K.L.; Ekhlaspour, L.; Sinha, M.; Mondesir, D.; Esmaeili, A.; Hartigan, C.; Thompson, M.J.; Malkani, S. Home use of a bihormonal bionic pancreas versus insulin pump therapy in adults with type 1 diabetes: A multicenter randomised crossover trial. *Lancet* **2017**, *389*, 369–380. [CrossRef]

57. Kovatchev, B.; Cobelli, C.; Renard, E.; Anderson, S.; Breton, M.; Patek, S.; Clarke, W.; Bruttomesso, D.; Maran, A.; Costa, S.; et al. Multinational study of subcutaneous model-predictive closed-loop control in type 1 diabetes mellitus: Summary of results. *J. Diabetes Sci. Technol.* **2010**, *4*, 1374–1381. [CrossRef]

58. Phillip, M.; Battelino, T.; Atlas, E.; Kordonouri, O.; Bratina, N.; Miller, S.; Biester, T.; Stefanija, M.A.; Muller, I.; Nimri, R.; et al. Nocturnal glucose control with an artificial pancreas at a diabetes camp. *N. Engl. J. Med.* **2013**, *368*, 824–833. [CrossRef]

59. Kovatchev, B.P.; Renard, E.; Cobelli, C.; Zisser, H.C.; Keith-Hynes, P.; Anderson, S.M.; Brown, S.A.; Chernavvsky, D.R.; Breton, M.D.; et al. Safety of outpatient closed-loop control: First randomized crossover trials of a wearable artificial pancreas. *Diabetes Care* **2014**, *37*, 1789–1796. [CrossRef]

60. Trevitt, S.; Simpson, S.; Wood, A. Artificial pancreas device systems for the closed-loop control of type 1 diabetes: What systems are in development? *J. Diabetes Sci. Technol.* **2016**, *10*, 714–723. [CrossRef]

61. U.S. Food & Drug Administration. Summary of Safety and Effectiveness Data (SSED) of the Medtronic MiniMed 670G System (2016). Available online: www.accessdata.fda.gov/cdrhdocs/pdf16/P160017b.pdf (accessed on 3 March 2019).

62. Stone, J.Y.; Haviland, N.; Bailey, T.S. Review of a commercially available hybrid closed-loop insulin-delivery system in the treatment of type 1 diabetes. *Ther. Deliv.* **2018**, *9*, 77–87. [CrossRef]

63. Buckingham, B.A.; Forlenza, G.P.; Pinsker, J.E.; Christiansen, M.P.; Wadwa, R.P.; Schneider, J.; Peyser, T.A.; Dassau, E.; Lee, J.B.; O'Conner, J.; et al. Safety and Feasibility of the OmniPod Hybrid Closed-Loop System in Adult, Adolescent, and Pediatric Patients with Type 1 Diabetes Using a Personalized Model Predictive Control Algorithm. *Diabetes Technol. Ther.* **2018**, *20*, 257–262. [CrossRef]

64. Tandem Diabetes Care. Available online: http://investor.tandemdiabetes.com/news-releases/news-release-details/tandem-diabetes-care-and-typezero-technologies-announce-license (accessed on 10 March 2019).

65. Brown, S.; Raghinaru, D.; Emory, E.; Kovatchev, B. First Look at Control-IQ: A New-Generation Automated Insulin Delivery System. *Diabetes Care* **2018**, *41*, 2634–2636. [CrossRef]

66. Weaver, K.W.; Hirsch, I.B. The Hybrid Closed-Loop System: Evolution and Practical Applications. *Diabetes Technol. Ther.* **2018**, *20* (Suppl. 2), S216–S223. [CrossRef]

67. Bekiari, E.; Kitsios, K.; Thabit, H.; Tauschmann, M.; Athanasiadou, E.; Karagiannis, T.; Haidich, A.B.; Hovorka, R.; Tsapas, A. Artificial pancreas treatment for outpatients with type 1 diabetes: Systematic review and meta-analysis. *BMJ* **2018**, *361*, k1310. [CrossRef]

68. Cameron, F.M.; Ly, T.T.; Buckingham, B.A.; Maahs, D.M.; Forlenza, G.P.; Levy, C.J.; Lam, D.; Clinton, P.; Messer, L.H.; Westfall, E.; et al. Closed-loop control without meal announcement in type 1 diabetes. *Diabetes Technol. Ther.* **2017**, *19*, 527–532. [CrossRef]

69. Forlenza, G.P.; Cameron, F.M.; Ly, T.T.; Lam, D.; Howsmon, D.P.; Baysal, N.; Kulina, G.; Messer, L.; Clinton, P.; Levister, C.; et al. Fully closed-loop multiple model probabilistic predictive controller artificial pancreas performance in adolescents and adults in the supervised hotel setting. *Diabetes Technol. Ther.* **2018**, *20*, 335–343. [CrossRef]

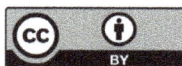

Review

Pediatric Sarcoidosis: A Review with Emphasis on Early Onset and High-Risk Sarcoidosis and Diagnostic Challenges

Brian Chiu [1,*], Jackie Chan [1], Sumit Das [1,2], Zainab Alshamma [1] and Consolato Sergi [1,3]

1   Department of Laboratory Medicine and Pathology, University of Alberta, Edmonton, Alberta T6G 2B7, Canada; jackiech@ualberta.ca (J.C.); sumit1@ualberta.ca (S.D.); zalshamm@ualberta.ca (Z.A.); sergi@ualberta.ca (C.S.)
2   Section of Neuropathology, University of Alberta, Edmonton, Alberta T6G 2B7, Canada
3   Department of Paediatrics, University of Alberta, Edmonton, Alberta T6G 2B7, Canada
*   Correspondence: bchiu@ualberta.ca; Tel.: +1-780-407-6959

Received: 15 August 2019; Accepted: 21 October 2019; Published: 25 October 2019

Abstract: Sarcoidosis is a non-necrotizing granulomatous inflammatory syndrome with multisystemic manifestations. We performed a systematic review of sarcoidosis in the pediatric population with particular emphases on early onset sarcoidosis, high-risk sarcoidosis, and newly reported or unusual sarcoid-related diseases. Blau Syndrome and early onset sarcoidosis/ BS-EOS are seen in children younger than five years old presenting with extra-thoracic manifestations but usually without lymphadenopathy and/or pulmonary involvement. The prevalence of high-risk sarcoidosis is very low in children and is further limited by the difficulty of diagnosis in symptomatic children and underdiagnosis in subclinical or asymptomatic patients. Reports of sarcoidal syndromes in users of E-cigarette/marijuana/other flavorings and their induction in cancer immunotherapies are of interests and may be challenging to differentiate from metastatic malignancy. The diagnostic considerations in pediatric sarcoidosis are to support a compatible clinicoradiographic presentation and the pathologic findings of non-necrotizing granulomas by ruling out granulomas of infective etiology. There is no absolutely reliable diagnostic test for sarcoidosis at present. The use of endoscopic bronchial ultrasound (EBUS) and transbronchial fine needle aspiration (TBNA) sampling of intrathoracic lymph nodes and lung, and for superficially accessible lesions, with cytopathological assessment and pathological confirmations provide fair diagnostic yield and excellent patient safety profile in children.

Keywords: Paediatric sarcoidosis; high-risk sarcoidosis; early-onset sarcoidosis; diagnostics; Blau syndrome

---

1. Introduction

Sarcoidosis is a multisystemic syndrome with a highly variable clinical course and diverse disease manifestations [1]. The incidence of sarcoidosis in adults may be biphasic [2]. Historically, it was thought to commonly affect young adults 30–50 years of age, but recent studies have reported that more than half of incident diagnoses are made in patients over 55 years of age [2,3]. Erdal and others suggest that the rates of sarcoidosis are increasing [4]. Approximately 25% of affected individuals with the disease develop chronic and progressive disease, which contributes to increased disease burden [5,6]. The mortality rate also appears to be rising [7]. There is no single diagnostic test for sarcoidosis. Instead, the diagnosis relies on specific pathologic and radiographic features in the appropriate clinical settings. The disease is characterized by pathologic findings of non-necrotizing granulomas in one or more involved organ systems after alternative diagnoses, in particular, infective etiologies, have been entertained [8].

Sarcoidosis is an ever-evolving process. The clinical phenotypes range from single-organ, self-limited, asymptomatic disease to multi-organ involvement with high-risk manifestations [9]. Hilar lymphadenopathy and pulmonary interstitial infiltrations are the most common manifestations [10]. The term "high-risk sarcoidosis" was introduced at the National Heart Lung and Blood Institute Sarcoidosis Workshop 2017 [1] to denote several manifestations of sarcoidosis that are associated with impaired quality of life and relatively high risk of death [9]. These include treatment-resistant pulmonary sarcoidosis, cardiac sarcoidosis, neurosarcoidosis, and/or multi-organ involvement. The high-risk manifestations and multi-organ involvements are often missed until late in the disease course [9].

The diagnosis of sarcoidosis is relatively uncommon in children [8,11–13], and high-risk sarcoid may present differently in children than in adults [8,14]. In this review, we search the English literature and aim to review the clinical investigations and laboratory diagnostics of sarcoidosis in this population.

2. Materials and Methods

We performed a systematic narrative review on sarcoidosis with particular emphases on early onset sarcoidosis, high-risk sarcoidosis, and newly reported or unusual sarcoid-related diseases in the pediatric population. We searched PubMed, Scopus, Google Scholars, and Cochrane Database of Systematic Reviews, using the following terms: sarcoidosis, pediatric, juvenile, children; high-risk sarcoidosis; pulmonary sarcoidosis; treatment-resistant sarcoidosis; cardiac sarcoid; and neurosarcoidosis. We also searched references from the appropriate reviews and case reports.

3. Results

The true incidence and prevalence of sarcoidosis in children is unknown as the disease is much less common in children than in adults [13]. It is difficult to diagnose in symptomatic children and may remain undiagnosed in subclinical or asymptomatic patients [8,11]. Several larger reviews reported that the incidence of clinically recognized sarcoidosis in children was 0.22 to 0.29/100,000 children per year, and gradually increases with age to a small peak in teenagers at 13–15 years of age [2,8,11,13,15]. Two distinct forms of childhood sarcoidosis appear to exist. Older children and young adults present most frequently with a multisystemic disease in a combination of lymphadenopathy, pulmonary, ocular and cutaneous involvement (erythema nodosum) [2,8,11,13], followed by joint (sarcoidal arthritis) and hepatosplenic features [8,11,13]. The disease patterns and clinical outcomes are similar to those in adults.

3.1. Blau Syndrome and Early Onset Sarcoidosis (BS-EOS)

In younger children, the majority of cases of EOS seen in children younger than five years old uniquely presents with a clinical triad of uveitis, arthritis, and skin rash [2]. In 1985, Blau et al. reported a rare autosomal dominant inflammatory disease characterized by a clinical triad of granulomatous dermatitis, recurrent granulomatous uveitis, and systemic polyarthritis in 11 family members of four generations [16,17]. A mutation of nucleotide binding oligomerization domain 2 (NOD2), also termed caspase recruitment domain–containing protein 15 (CARD15), mapped on chromosome 16q12 was identified [18] and found to be responsible for these granulomatous inflammations [16,18]. Early onset sarcoidosis (EOS) is caused by a sporadic mutation of the NOD2 gene, with similar clinical manifestations to Blau Syndrome [16]. Blau Syndrome/EOS patients rarely present with pulmonary involvement, and ocular involvement tends to follow prior articular and cutaneous manifestations in these patients [16,19].

CARD15/NOD2 encodes a multidomain cytosolic protein and is expressed primarily in the cytosol of antigen-presenting cells [20]. Stimulation by bacterial or viral infection [21] may promote the activation of nuclear factor kappa-light-chain-enhancer of activated B cells (NF-κB) and tumor necrosis factor receptor-associated factor 3 (TRAF3) signaling pathways [21]. A possible role of mycobacterial components has also been suggested as triggers of granulomatous autoinflammation in

CARD15/NOD2 mutations in BS/EOS [22–24]. Crohn's disease (CD) is a granulomatous inflammatory bowel disease, involving any part of the gastrointestinal tract [25] but may mainly affect the distal ileum and colon [22,26,27]. The CARD15/NOD2 gene has been identified as one of the genes linked to susceptibility to CD [22,28]. It has been hypothesized that NOD2 susceptibility loci in intestinal Paneth cells led to defective NF-κB activation, altered intestinal bacterial clearance and granulomatous inflammation [22,29,30]. Juvenile sarcoidosis presenting as Crohn's disease of the GIT has been reported [31].

3.2. High-Risk Sarcoidosis

Approximately 25% of affected individuals with sarcoidosis develop chronic or progressive disease [6]. Manifestations of sarcoidosis associated with poor prognosis and a relatively high risk of death include treatment-resistant pulmonary-, cardiac-, neuro-, and multiorgan sarcoidosis [9]. Pulmonary disease is the most common cause of chronic disease and death in adults [9]. As in adults, older children usually present with hilar lymphadenopathy and up to 50% present with interstitial lung disease and multiorgan involvement, while progression to chronic diseases occurs in 12% of these children [2,8,13]. Korsten et al. defined pulmonary sarcoidosis refractory to treatment as progressive disease and significant impairment of life despite glucocorticoid therapy for at least three months and the need for additional anti-sarcoid drugs [32]. These patients develop progressive pulmonary fibrosis and associated complications, including pulmonary hypertension and infections and are seen in more than 10% of patients at specialized centers [32,33]. In infants and children younger than five years, the typical pulmonary diseases are usually not seen [8]. In a retrospective study of 41 pediatric patients, which were followed for 18 months on disease presentation, management, and clinical outcome, those patients with pulmonary sarcoidosis diagnosed before 10 years old were more likely to recover and presented with fewer relapses compared with the patients diagnosed after 10 years old [34].

Recent progress in cell-mediated immunity and granuloma formation has advanced our understanding of the development of sarcoidosis [8,35]. Macrophages bearing increased expression of major histocompatibility (MHC) class II molecules, different subsets of T-lymphocytes and other immune effector cells such as mast cells and natural killer cells may be at play [8,35]. In sarcoidosis involving the lung, before the formation of granulomas, early lesions consist of alveolitis with a high proportion of activated CD4+ T-cells [36]. T-cells play a role in amplification of the local cellular immune response and are responsible for secretion of cytokines, including tumor necrosis factor (TNF), which favors granulomatous response at the sites of disease activity. The diagnostic approach to pulmonary sarcoidosis has been revolutionized in the past decade by the use of endobronchial ultrasound (EBUS) real-time guided transbronchial sampling of intrathoracic lymph nodes and lung biopsies [6]. Cytopathological assessments by fine needle aspiration provide fair diagnostic yield and excellent patient safety profile in children [37,38]. Combining EBUS and transbronchial needle aspiration (TBNA) lung biopsy and cytopathologic study may increase the diagnostic sensitivity to close to 100% [39,40]. On bronchoalveolar lavage (BAL) fluid with lymphocytosis (15%) and increased ratio of CD4 to CD8 (>3.5:1), the specificity for the diagnosis of sarcoidosis approaches 95% [36,41].

Cardiac sarcoidosis (CS) is a rare but potentially fatal condition [42]. Clinically recognizable cardiac involvement occurs in 5% of adult patients with sarcoidosis [43], and granulomatous inflammation of the heart was recognized in up to 25% in an autopsy series [13,44]. Rare cases of pediatric cardiac sarcoidosis had been reported [8]. Patients with CS may present with a wide variety of signs and symptoms, ranging from asymptomatic ECG abnormalities to sudden death [42]. Congestive heart failure and conduction abnormalities are the two most common clinical manifestations in CS [42], with one case presenting with pericardial effusion [2,8]. Many patients with pulmonary/systemic sarcoidosis have asymptomatic cardiac involvement [43]. A high index of suspicion and early diagnosis are crucial when immunosuppression therapy may result in reduced mortality rate [8]. Various imaging modalities including echocardiography and/or CMR imaging may be utilized [43].

Neurosarcoidosis occurs in fewer than 5% of adult with systemic sarcoid with isolated neurosarcoidosis being more rare [45], and to our knowledge, 53 cases of pediatric neurosarcoidosis have been reported in the English literature [14,46]. In these children, the most common manifestations include headache, seizures, cranial neuropathy, optic neuritis, and hypothalamic and/or pituitary dysfunction [14,46]. Compared to the adult counterparts, prepubertal children with neurosarcoidosis are more likely to present with seizures and a space-occupying lesion but less likely with cranial nerve palsies. These children do however tend to evolve to an adult pattern of presentation during puberty [14]. Single cases of aqueductal stenosis [13] and obstructive hydrocephalus [47] have also been reported. The most reliable method for diagnosing neurosarcoidosis is via biopsy of lesion in the central nervous system revealing non-caseating granuloma [46]. Microscopically, granulomatous inflammation is typically found in the meninges, ventricles (including choroid plexus) and adjacent brain or spinal cord parenchyma. Inflammatory infiltrate may involve optic nerve and chiasm, cranial nerves such as facial, auditory, and vestibulocochlear nerve. In cases where biopsy is not possible, neuroimaging becomes an important diagnostic modality. The most common neuroimaging finding is said to be leptomeningeal enhancement on T1-weighted MRI with contrast administration [48]. Enhancement may also be seen in the basilar region, leading to abnormalities in the hypothalamus, optic chiasm, and pituitary region [46]. As neurosarcoidosis is a diagnosis of exclusion, differential diagnoses that need to be considered and ruled out include tuberculosis, fungus, Wegener's granulomatosis and hypertrophic meningitis, as these may also present with leptomeningeal enhancement and granulomas. To the best of our knowledge, cases of pediatric spinal neurosarcoidosis have not been reported in the English literature.

3.3. Acute Sarcoidosis

In contrast to the chronic progressive disease with organ dysfunction in high-risk sarcoidosis, two acute sarcoidosis syndromes are of relatively benign clinical outcome. Lofgren syndrome is characterized by fever, bilateral hilar lymphadenopathy, erythema nodosum, and arthralgia, typically in young women, primarily Caucasian. Prognosis is excellent with complete resolution of the disease in 90% of the patients within two years [8,49,50]. Heerfordt syndrome or uveoparotid fever, presenting with a combination of fever, parotidomegaly, anterior uveitis, and cranial nerve palsy is usually seen in adults but has been reported in children [8,49]. The disease is normally self-limiting with cure achieved between 1–3 years [8,51]. The acute sarcoidosis syndromes may be confidently diagnosed on clinical grounds without surgical biopsy confirmation in adults [8,49,52]. However, the clinical manifestations in children may be variable necessitating biopsy histopathology confirmation [8,15,49,53].

Pathology images of the spectrum of pediatric sarcoidosis involving different organs (Figures 1–7).

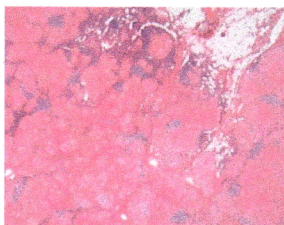

Figure 1. Mediastinal nodal sarcoidosis. H&E Magnification 20×.

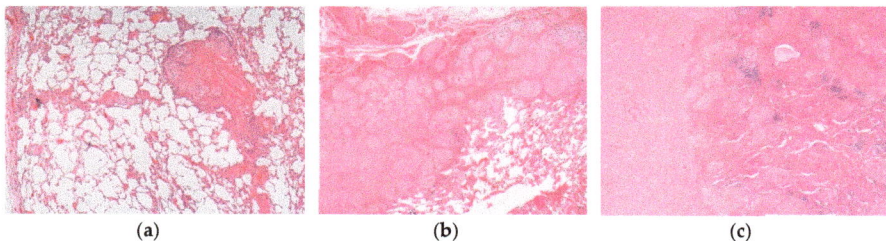

(a)   (b)   (c)

Figure 2. Pulmonary sarcoidosis. (**a**) Pulmonary sarcoidosis. (**b**) Pulmonary nodular sarcoidosis. (**c**) Pulmonary fibrotic sarcoidosis. H&E. Magnifications 20×, 50×.

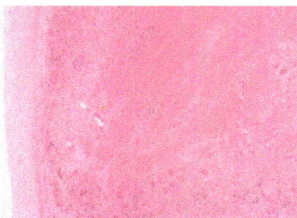

Figure 3. Cardiac sarcoidosis. H&E Magnification 50×.

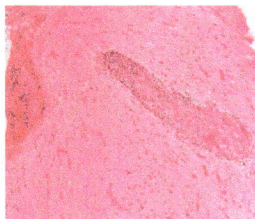

Figure 4. Neurosarcoidosis. H&E. Magnification 100×.

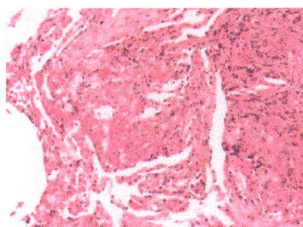

Figure 5. Lung sarcoidosis young E-cig vaper. H&E. Magnification 200×.

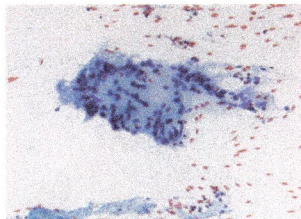

Figure 6. Acute sarcoidosis salivary gland. Cytopathology Pap stain 200×.

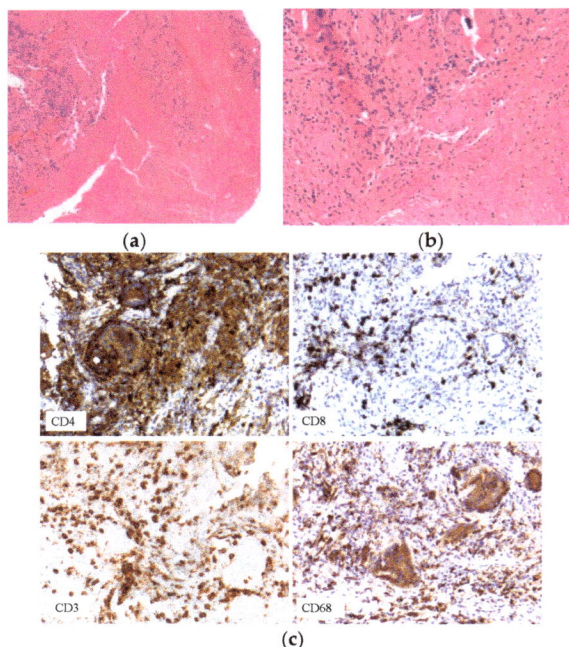

Figure 7. Immune cell phenotypes: T-cells: CD3, CD4, CD8; macrophage CD68. (**a**) Early onset sarcoidosis (EOS) skin sarcoidosis; (**b–c**) EOS skin sarcoidosis.

Recent case reports of sarcoidosis developing after antigen exposure to inhalation or in immune-therapy are of interests. The popularity of electronic cigarettes (E-cig) has recently been increasing among adolescents and young adults [54–56]. E-cig usage or "vaping" contains E-liquid carrier components, flavorings, and marijuana product with cannabidiol (CBD) formulations [57–60]. In anecdotal stories, the use of medical marijuana, in particular vaping with CBD oil may be linked to improvement of refractory pulmonary sarcoidosis [61]. In E-cig and marijuana users, sarcoidal granulomas are found in multiple organs in case reports, raising the clinical suspicion of metastatic malignancy [62,63]. The development of sarcoidal granulomas may be related to vaped marijuana product tetrahydrocannabinol (THC), E-cig flavorings, or contaminants. An association of vaped THC has been reportedly seen in close to 500 cases of severe pulmonary disease with six confirmed deaths [56]. As tumor necrosis factor-alpha (TNF-α) plays an important role in both formation and maintenance of sarcoidal granulomas, anti-TNF-α may provide a therapeutic option to patients with sarcoidosis [64]. However, many anti-TNF-associated cases of sarcoidosis have also been reported [65], negating its therapeutic usage. Pulmonary sarcoidal granulomas are found in patients undergoing interferon-alpha therapy [66]. The use of immune checkpoint inhibitors by enhancing anti-tumor immunity has revolutionized cancer therapy recently, and their use for cancer immunotherapy in pediatric patients may have potential benefits [67,68]. However, pulmonary sarcoidosis and the exacerbation of sarcoidosis leading to central nervous system involvement after immune checkpoint inhibitor therapy have been reported [25,69].

3.4. Diagnostic Challenges and Considerations in Pediatric Sarcoidosis

There is no absolutely reliable diagnostic test for sarcoidosis [52]. A number of clinical tests and biomarkers assay have evolved over time in the diagnosis and include: tubulin skin test of anergy (Kvim test), serum angiotensin-converting enzyme (SACE), serum amyloid A (SAA), and cytokine levels [33,52,70]. The lack of sensitivity and specificity of these tests or biomarkers poorly suited as screening tests, disease activity or prognostic markers for sarcoidosis [33,52,70]. As in adults, the diagnosis is difficult to confirm in symptomatic children, and there is a significant number of asymptomatic patients who remain undiagnosed [13].

In the spectrum of pediatric sarcoidosis, depending on the initial clinical presentation and subsequent investigations including various diagnostic imaging modalities, sarcoidosis is a diagnosis of exclusion, with ruling out granulomatous infections, in particular by Mycobacterial and fungal organisms [8,52]. A high index of suspicion is critical in the diagnosis, especially in early onset of the disease or Blau syndrome in a child younger than five years of age who presents with a clinical triad of uveitis, arthritis, and skin rash, and without the adult manifestations of lymphadenopathy and/or pulmonary involvement. The early presentation of arthritis in early onset sarcoidosis may be misdiagnosed as juvenile rheumatoid arthritis (JRA) [71]. Pediatric sarcoidosis involving the gastrointestinal tract may raise a differential diagnosis mostly with Crohn's disease [31]. Both sarcoidosis and CD are chronic granulomatous inflammatory disorders. The presence of granulomas in the gastrointestinal tract might be misleading and the diagnosis of sarcoidosis should be established when extraintestinal features become evident [31]. For BS/EOS and acute sarcoidosis syndromes, pathological and/or cytopathological confirmation and exclusion of other etiologies by biopsies of accessible lesions such as skin (including erythema nodosum, which is a non-granulomatous panniculitis) [49], salivary glands, and peripheral lymph nodes are highly desirable.

Cases of high-risk sarcoidosis in children with the involvement of treatment-resistant pulmonary disease, cardiac sarcoidosis, neurosarcoidosis, and multi-organ disease and the recent reports of E-cigarettes and immunotherapy-related sarcoidosis are uncommon. The lung is the most frequent site for biopsy confirmation, followed by skin, peripheral lymph nodes, and liver [49,72]. The diagnostic considerations are to support a compatible clinicoradiographic presentation and the demonstration of non-caseating granulomas. The use of EBUS-TBNA sampling of intrathoracic lymph nodes and lung [6], with cytopathological assessments and pathological confirmations provide fair diagnostic yield and excellent patient safety profile in children [6,52] (Figure 8).

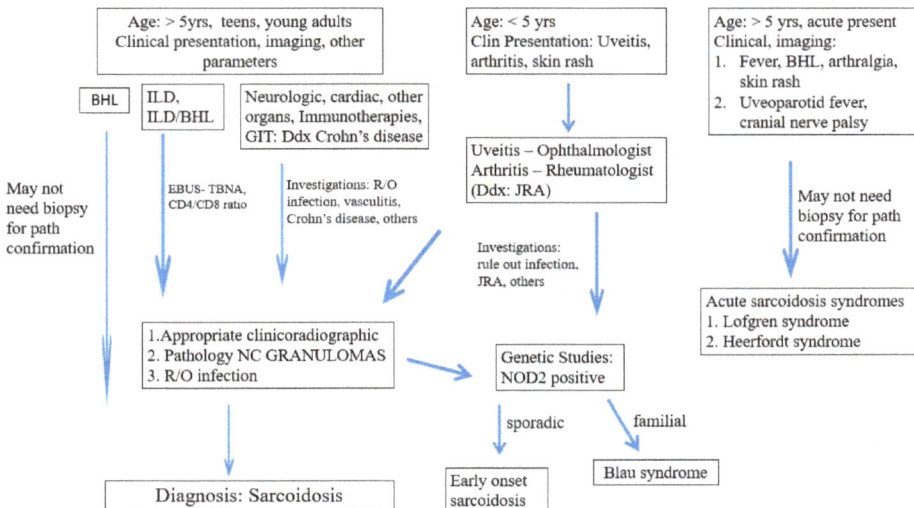

Figure 8. Paediatric Sarcoidosis: Diagnostic Considerations. Legends: BHL Bilateral hilar lymphadenopathy, ILD Interstitial lung disease, GIT gastrointestinal tract, EBUS-TBNA endoscopic bronchial ultrasound-transbronchial needle aspiration, NG non-necrotizing granulomas, JRA Juvenile rheumatoid arthritis, NOD2 Nucleotide binding oligomerization domain 2.

4. Discussions

Since the initial clinical description by Jonathan Hutchinson [73] in 1877, followed by the histologic findings of Caesar Boeck [74] in 1899, recent progress in immunology and molecular biology has advanced our understanding of the pathogenetic mechanisms for the development of sarcoidosis [8,35,75]. The proposed model of sarcoidal granuloma development in children involves the interplay of environmental triggers by a variety of antigens and immunologic/genetic/epigenetic factors, and requires three or more events to take place [8] (Figure 9)—environmental exposures to antigen (e.g., infectious agents, E-cigarettes flavorings, marijuana), acquired cellular immunity directed against the antigen, and the appearance of immune effector cells that promote a non-specific inflammatory response [8]. The subsequent Th1 (CD4+ T cell) polarized immune response with increased cytokine activities (TNF, IFNγ, interleukin) [75], and high-level IFNγ-secreting Th17 effector cells [35] are at play in the recruitment and proliferation of immune cells. Genetic factors (e.g., CARD15/ NOD2 mutation) may play a role by interacting with mycobacterial/bacterial/viral components, promoting the activation of NF-κB and tumor necrosis factor receptor-associated factor 3 (TRAF3) signaling pathways and triggering granulomatous autoinflammation in BS/EOS patients [22–24]. Immune checkpoint inhibitor (PD-1/PD-L1) for the immunotherapy of a variety of cancers may activate T-cells and promote granuloma formation [25,69]. Progression of granulomatous inflammation and putative antigen persistence promotes fibrosis and the development of high-risk organ-system manifestations [35,75].

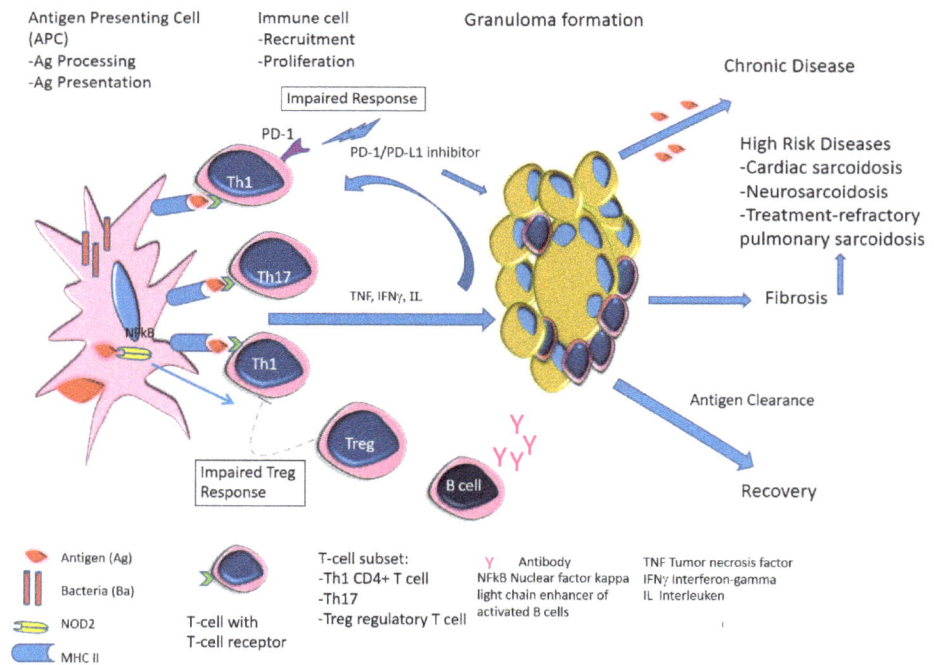

Figure 9. Proposed Pathogenetic Mechanisms in Pediatric Sarcoidosis.

Lofgren syndrome patients develop acute sarcoidosis, and show reduced frequency of lung-resident regulatory T cells (T-reg). The T-reg, however, super-synthesizes interleukin IL10, as supported by the detection of increased BAL fluid IL10 concentration [76], thus, creating an immunosuppressive micro-environment [35]. B lymphocytes may also be involved in sarcoidal granuloma formation, as Lofgren syndrome patients exhibit higher levels of Proprionibacterium acnes-specific IgA antibodies [77]. In chronic diseases, sarcoid T-reg fails to efficiently suppress proliferation and cytokine production by T helper cells [78], and with accumulation of Th1/Th17 cells, further support stabilization of granulomas and chronic disease progression [35]. In contrast, highly plastic and qualified effector T-cells aiming at clearance of the antigens from the granulomas leads to recovery [35,76].

We summarize the clinicopathologic spectrum of pediatric sarcoidosis and the diagnostic considerations in Table 1. Erdal and others suggest that the rates of adult sarcoidosis are increasing [4]. With the risks of increasing environmental exposure to increasing number of antigens, we would expect the prevalence of pediatric sarcoidosis also correspondingly increases. At present, there are no absolute diagnostic tests or biomarkers for screening, disease activity or prognostic markers for sarcoidosis. Fortunately, the diagnosis of sarcoidosis in children is improving with ever improving diagnostic techniques and imaging modalities. The development of minimally invasive procedures including EBUS-TBNA, for cytopathology or pathological confirmation of non-necrotizing granulomas and the resultant improving prognosis outcome appear promising. Recent advances in the use of genome-based approaches in identifying novel biomarkers to support the diagnosis and predict disease activity yield some promising results [70]. However, further researches are needed in sarcoidosis involving the young population.

Table 1. Pediatric sarcoidosis—clinicopathologic spectrum.

Entity	Clinical	Laboratory	Pathology	References
-Prevalence -Systems involved -Prognosis	-0.22–0.29/10^6 -Lymph nodes/Lung -Chronic disease 12%	BAL: CD4/CD8 Biopsies	Granulomas Figure 1	[2,8,11,13,15]
-Early-onset sarcoidosis/ Blau syndrome	Triad: uveitis, arthritis, skin rash	Eye exam Biopsy	Granulomas Figure 7	[22,23,79]
High-risk sarcoid -Treatment-resistant Pulmonary sarcoid	-Most common, progression to chronicity	Chest XR, CT, EBUS/TBNA	Figure 2	[2,9,13]; [2,6,8,14,34,46]
-Cardiac sarcoid/CS -Neurosarcoid/ NS	-CS Case reports -NS 53 cases	Cardiac echo CT /MRI	Figure 3 Figure 4	
Sarcoid-like syndrome -INF therapy -Checkpoint inhibitor -E-cig/Marijuana	-Not reported in children -Not reported in children -Teens and young adults	Imaging modalities Biopsy	Figure 5	[66] [25,69]; [62,63]
Acute sarcoidosis -Lofgren syndrome -Heerfordt syndrome /uveoparotid fever	Triad: erythema nodosum BHL (CXR), arthritis, Resolution in two years Uveitis, parotidomegaly, facial nerve palsy, fever, Prognosis excellent	Chest XR, CT, biopsy	Both can be Diagnosed on clinical data without biopsy Figure 6	[50]; [8,49]

BAL bronchoalveolar lavage, EBUS endoscopic transbronchial ultrasound biopsy, TBNA transbronchial needle aspiration, IFNα interferon-alpha therapy, CPI checkpoint inhibitor therapy, Electronic-cigarette E-cig, BHL (CXR) bilateral hilar lymphadenopathy on chest X-ray.

Author Contributions: The authors' contributions are as follows: conceptualization, B.C. and C.S.; methodology, B.C.; software, B.C., and J.C.; validation, B.C., C.S., J.C., S.D. and Z.A.; formal analysis, B.C.; investigation, B.C., C.S.; resources, B.C.; data curation, B.C. and J.C.; writing—original draft preparation, B.C.; writing—review and editing, B.C., J.C., S.D. and C.S.; visualization, B.C.; supervision, B.C. and C.S.; project administration, B.C.

Funding: This research received no external funding

Conflicts of Interest: The authors declare no conflict of interest.

References

1. Maier, L.A.; Crouser, E.D.; Martin, W.J., II; Eu, J. Executive Summary of the NHLBI Workshop Report: Leveraging Current Scientific Advancements to Understand Sarcoidosis Variability and Improve Outcomes. *Ann. Am. Thorac. Soc.* **2017**, *14*, S415–S420. [CrossRef] [PubMed]
2. Gedalia, A.; Khan, T.A.; Shetty, A.K.; Dimitriades, V.R.; Espinoza, L.R. Childhood sarcoidosis: Louisiana experience. *Clin. Rheumatol.* **2016**, *35*, 1879–1884. [CrossRef] [PubMed]
3. Levin, A.M.; Iannuzzi, M.C.; Montgomery, C.G.; Trudeau, S.; Datta, I.; McKeigue, P.; Fischer, A.; Nebel, A.; Rybicki, B.A. Association of ANXA11 genetic variation with sarcoidosis in African Americans and European Americans. *Genes Immun.* **2013**, *14*, 13–18. [CrossRef] [PubMed]
4. Erdal, B.S.; Clymer, B.D.; Yildiz, V.O.; Julian, M.W.; Crouser, E.D. Unexpectedly high prevalence of sarcoidosis in a representative U.S. Metropolitan population. *Respir. Med.* **2012**, *106*, 893–899. [CrossRef]
5. Gerke, A.K.; Judson, M.A.; Cozier, Y.C.; Culver, D.A.; Koth, L.L. Disease Burden and Variability in Sarcoidosis. *Ann. Am. Thorac. Soc.* **2017**, *14*, S421–S428. [CrossRef]
6. Spagnolo, P.; Rossi, G.; Trisolini, R.; Sverzellati, N.; Baughman, R.P.; Wells, A.U. Pulmonary sarcoidosis. *Lancet Respir. Med.* **2018**, *6*, 389–402. [CrossRef]
7. Swigris, J.J.; Oison, A.; Huie, T.J.; Fernandez-Perez, E.R.; Solomon, J.; Sprunger, D.; Brown, K.K. Sarcoidosis-related mortality in the United States from 1988 to 2007. *Am. J. Respir. Crit. Care Med.* **2011**, *183*, 1524–1530. [CrossRef]
8. Shetty, A.K.; Gedalia, A. Sarcoidosis in children. *Curr. Probl. Pediatr.* **2000**, *30*, 149–176. [CrossRef]
9. Sauer, W.H.; Stern, B.J.; Baughman, R.P.; Culver, D.A.; Royal, W. High-Risk Sarcoidosis. Current Concepts and Research Imperatives. *Ann. Am. Thorac. Soc.* **2017**, *14*, S437–S444. [CrossRef]
10. Neville, E.; Walker, A.N.; James, D.G. Prognostic factors predicting the outcome of sarcoidosis: An analysis of 818 patients. *QJM Int. J. Med.* **1983**, *52*, 525–533.
11. Hoffmann, A.L.; Milman, N.; Byg, K.E. Childhood sarcoidosis in Denmark 1979–1994: Incidence, clinical features and laboratory results at presentation in 48 children. *Acta Paediatr.* **2004**, *93*, 30–36. [CrossRef] [PubMed]
12. Hunninghake, G.W.; Costabel, U.; Ando, M.; Baughman, R.; Cordier, J.F.; du Bois, R.; Eklund, A.; Kitaichi, M.; Lynch, J.; Rizzato, G.; et al. ATS/ERS/WASOG statement on sarcoidosis. American Thoracic Society/European Respiratory Society/World Association of Sarcoidosis and other Granulomatous Disorders. *Sarcoidosis Vasc. Diffus. Lung Dis.* **1999**, *16*, 149–173.
13. Pattishall, E.N.; Kending, E.J. Sarcoidosis in children. *Pediatr. Pulmonol.* **1996**, *22*, 195–203. [CrossRef]
14. Baumann, R.J.; Robertson, W.C. Neurosarcoid presents differently in children than in adults. *Pediatrics* **2003**, *112*, e480–e486. [CrossRef] [PubMed]
15. Milman, N.; Hoffmann, A.; Byg, K.E. Sarcoidosis in children. Epidemiology in Danes, clinical features, diagnosis, treatment and prognosis. *Acta Paediatr.* **1998**, *87*, 871–878. [CrossRef] [PubMed]
16. Achille, M.; Ilaria, P.; Teresa, G.; Roberto, C.; Ilir, A.; Piergiorgio, N.; Rolando, C.; Gabriele, S. Successful treatment with adalimumab for severe multifocal choroiditis and panuveitis in presumed (early-onset) ocular sarcoidosis. *Int. Ophthalmol.* **2016**, *36*, 129–135. [CrossRef] [PubMed]
17. Blau, E.B. Familial granulomatous arthritis, iritis, and rash. *J. Pediatr.* **1985**, *107*, 689–693. [CrossRef]
18. Miceli-Richard, C.; Lesage, S.; Rybojad, M.; Prieur, A.M.; Manouvrier-Hanu, S.; Häfner, R.; Chamaillard, M.; Zouali, H.; Thomas, G.; Hugot, J.P. CARD15 mutations in Blau syndrome. *Nat. Genet.* **2001**, *29*, 19–20. [CrossRef]
19. Rosé, C.D.; Aróstegui, J.; Martin, T.M.; Espada, G.; Scalzi, L.; Yagüe, J.; Rosenbaum, J.T.; Modesto, C.; Cristina Arnal, M.; Merino, R.; et al. NOD2-associated pediatric granulomatous arthritis, an expanding phenotype: Study of an international registry and a national cohort in Spain. *Arthritis Rheum.* **2009**, *60*, 1797–1803. [CrossRef]
20. Philpott, D.J.; Sorbara, M.; Robertson, S.J.; Croitoru, K.; Girardin, S.E. NOD proteins: Regulators of inflammation in health and disease. *Nat. Rev. Immunol.* **2014**, *14*, 9–23. [CrossRef]
21. Moreira, L.O.; Zamboni, D. NOD1 and NOD2 Signaling in Infection and Inflammation. *Front. Immunol.* **2012**, *3*, 328. [CrossRef] [PubMed]

22. Caso, F.; Galozzi, P.; Costa, L.; Sfriso, P.; Cantarini, L.; Punzi, L. Autoinflammatory granulomatous diseases: From Blau syndrome and early-onset sarcoidosis to NOD2-mediated disease and Crohn's disease. *RMD Open* **2015**, *1*, e000097. [CrossRef] [PubMed]

23. Caso, F.; Wouters, C.; Rose, C.D.; Costa, L.; Tognon, S.; Sfriso, P.; Cantarini, L.; Rigante, D.; Punzi, L. Blau syndrome and latent tubercular infection: An unresolved partnership. *Int. J. Rheum. Dis.* **2014**, *17*, 586–587. [CrossRef] [PubMed]

24. Dow, C.T.; Ellingson, J. Detection of Mycobacterium avium ss. Paratuberculosis in Blau Syndrome Tissues. *Autoimmune Dis.* **2010**, *2011*, 127692. [CrossRef] [PubMed]

25. Noguchi, S.; Kawachi, H.; Yoshida, H.; Fukao, A.; Terashita, S.; Ikeue, T.; Horikawa, S.; Sugita, T. Sarcoid-Like Granulomatosis Induced by Nivolumab Treatment in a Lung Cancer Patient. *Case Rep. Oncol.* **2018**, *11*, 562–566. [CrossRef] [PubMed]

26. Abraham, C.; Cho, J.H. Inflammatory bowel disease. *N. Engl. J. Med.* **2009**, *36*, 2066–2078. [CrossRef]

27. Baumgart, D.C.; Sandborn, W. Crohn's disease. *Lancet* **2012**, *380*, 1590–1605. [CrossRef]

28. Ogura, Y.; Bonen, D.; Inohara, N.; Nicolae, D.L.; Chen, F.F.; Ramos, R.; Britton, H.; Moran, T.; Karaliuskas, R.; Duerr, R.H.; et al. A frameshift mutation in NOD2 associated with susceptibility to Crohn's disease. *Nature* **2001**, *411*, 603–606. [CrossRef]

29. Abraham, C.; Cho, J. Functional consequences of NOD2 (CARD15) mutations. *Inflamm. Bowel Dis.* **2006**, *12*, 641–650. [CrossRef]

30. Khor, B.; Gardet, A.; Xavier, R.J. Genetics and pathogenesis of inflammatory bowel disease. *Nature* **2011**, *474*, 307–317. [CrossRef]

31. Brunner, J.; Sergi, C.; Müller, T.; Gassner, I.; Prüfer, F.; Zimmerhackl, L.B. Juvenile sarcoidosis presenting as Crohn's disease. *Eur. J. Pediatr.* **2006**, *165*, 398–401. [CrossRef] [PubMed]

32. Korsten, P.; Strohmayer, K.; Baughman, R.P.; Sweiss, N.J. Refractory pulmonary sarcoidosis—Proposal of a definition and recommendations for the diagnostic and therapeutic approach. *Clin. Pulm. Med.* **2016**, *23*, 67–75. [CrossRef] [PubMed]

33. Baughman, R.P.; Culver, D.; Judson, M.A. A concise review of pulmonary sarcoidosis. *Am. J. Respir. Crit. Care Med.* **2011**, *183*, 573–581. [CrossRef]

34. Nathan, N.; Marcelo, P.; Houdouin, V.; Epaud, R.; de Blic, J.; Valeyre, D.; Houzel, A.; Busson, P.F.; Corvol, H.; Deschildre, A.; et al. Lung sarcoidosis in children: Update on disease expression and management. *Thorax* **2015**, *70*, 537–542. [CrossRef] [PubMed]

35. Sakthivel, P.; Bruder, D. Mechanism of granuloma formation in sarcoidosis. *Curr. Opin. Hematol.* **2017**, *24*, 59–65. [CrossRef] [PubMed]

36. Poulter, L.W.; Rossi, G.; Bjermer, L.; Costabel, U.; Israel-Biet, D.; Klech, H.; Pohl, W.; Velluti, G. The value of bronchoalveolar lavage in the diagnosis and prognosis of sarcoidosis. *Eur. Respir. J.* **1990**, *3*, 943–944.

37. Gulla, K.M.; Gunathilaka, G.; Jat, K.R.; Sankar, J.; Karan, M.; Lodha, R.; Kabra, S.K. Utility and safety of endobronchial ultrasound-guided transbronchial needle aspiration and endoscopic ultrasound with an echobronchoscope-guided fine needle aspiration in children with mediastinal pathology. *Pediatr. Pulmonol.* **2019**, *54*, 881–885. [CrossRef] [PubMed]

38. Sergi, C.; Dhiman, A.; Gray, J.A. Fine Needle Aspiration Cytology for Neck Masses in Childhood. An Illustrative Approach. *Diagnostics* **2018**, *8*, 28. [CrossRef]

39. Aragaki-Nakahodo, A.A.; Baughman, R.; Shipley, R.T.; Benzaquen, S. The complimentary role of transbronchial lung cryobiopsy and endobronchial ultrasound fine needle aspiration in the diagnosis of sarcoidosis. *Respir. Med.* **2017**, *131*, 65–69. [CrossRef]

40. Trisolini, R.; Bauqhman, R.; Spagnolo, P.; Culver, D.A. Endobronchial ultrasound-guided transbronchial needle aspiration in sarcoidosis: Beyond the diagnostic yield. *Respirology* **2019**, *24*, 531–542. [CrossRef]

41. Drent, M.; Mansour, K.; Linssen, C. Bronchoalveolar lavage in sarcoidosis. *Semin. Respir. Crit. Care Med.* **2007**, *28*, 486–495. [CrossRef] [PubMed]

42. Kim, J.S.; Judson, M.; Donnino, R.; Gold, M.; Cooper, L.T., Jr.; Prystowsky, E.N.; Prystowsky, S. Cardiac sarcoidosis. *Am. Heart J.* **2009**, *157*, 9–21. [CrossRef] [PubMed]

43. Birnie, D.H.; Nery, P.; Ha, A.C.; Beanlands, R.S. Cardiac Sarcoidosis. *J. Am. Coll. Cardiol.* **2016**, *68*, 411–421. [CrossRef] [PubMed]

44. Perry, A.; Vuitch, F. Causes of death in patients with sarcoidosis. A morphologic study of 38 autopsies with clinicopathologic correlations. *Arch. Pathol. Lab. Med.* **1995**, *119*, 167–172. [PubMed]

45. Nowak, D.A.; Widenka, D. Neurosarcoidosis: A review of its intracranial manifestation. *J. Neurol.* **2001**, *248*, 363–372. [CrossRef] [PubMed]

46. Rao, R.; Dimitriades, V.; Weimer, M.; Sandlin, C. Neurosarcoidosis in Pediatric Patients: A Case Report and Review of Isolated and Systemic Neurosarcoidosis. *Pediatr. Neurol.* **2016**, *63*, 45–52. [CrossRef]

47. Kendig, E.L. The clinical picture of sarcoidosis in children. *Pediatrics* **1974**, *54*, 289–292.

48. Lury, K.M.; Smith, J.; Matheus, M.G.; Castillo, M. Neurosarcoidosis–review of imaging findings. *Semin. Roentgenol.* **2004**, *39*, 495–504. [CrossRef]

49. Culver, D.A. Sarcoidosis. *Immunol. Allergy Clin. N. Am.* **2012**, *32*, 487–511. [CrossRef]

50. Lofgren, S.; Lundbäck, H. The bilateral hilar lymphoma syndrome; a study of the relation to tuberculosis and sarcoidosis in 212 cases. *Acta Med. Scand.* **1952**, *142*, 265–273. [CrossRef]

51. Fraga, R.C.; Kakizaki, P.; Valente, N.Y.S.; Portocarrero, L.K.L.; Teixeira, M.F.S.; Senise, P.F. Do you know this syndrome? Heerfordt-Waldenström syndrome. *An. Bras. Dermatol.* **2017**, *92*, 571–572. [CrossRef] [PubMed]

52. Govender, P.; Berman, J. The Diagnosis of Sarcoidosis. *Clin. Chest Med.* **2015**, *36*, 585–602. [CrossRef] [PubMed]

53. Shetty, A.K.; Gedalia, A. Childhood sarcoidosis: A rare but fascinating disorder. *Pediatr. Rheumatol.* **2008**, *23*, 16. [CrossRef] [PubMed]

54. Agaku, I.T.; Ayo-Yusuf, O.A.; Vardavas, C.I.; Connolly, G. Predictors and patterns of cigarette and smokeless tobacco use among adolescents in 32 countries, 2007–2011. *J. Adolesc. Health* **2014**, *54*, 47–53. [CrossRef] [PubMed]

55. Dutra, L.M.; Glantz, S. Electronic cigarettes and conventional cigarette use among U.S. adolescents: A cross-sectional study. *JAMA Pediatr.* **2014**, *168*, 610–617. [CrossRef] [PubMed]

56. Grégoire, M.C. Vaping risks for youth continue to emerge. *Can. Med. Assoc. J.* **2019**, *191*, E1113–E1114. [CrossRef] [PubMed]

57. Harrell, M.B.; Weaver, S.; Loukas, A.; Creamer, M.; Marti, C.N.; Jackson, C.D.; Heath, J.W.; Navak, P.; Perry, C.L.; Pechacek, T.F.; et al. Flavored e-cigarette use: Characterizing youth, young adult, and adult users. *Prev. Med. Rep.* **2016**, *11*, 33–40. [CrossRef]

58. Leigh, N.J.; Lawton, R.; Hershberger, P.A.; Goniewicz, M.L. Flavourings significantly affect inhalation toxicity of aerosol generated from electronic nicotine delivery systems (ENDS). *Tob. Control* **2016**, *25*, ii81–ii87. [CrossRef]

59. Tierney, P.A.; Karpinski, C.; Brown, J.E.; Luo, W.; Pankow, J.F. Flavour chemicals in electronic cigarette fluids. *Tob. Control* **2016**, *25*, e10–e15. [CrossRef]

60. Peace, M.R.; Butler, K.; Wolf, C.E.; Poklis, J.L.; Poklis, A. Evaluation of Two Commercially Available Cannabidiol Formulations for Use in Electronic Cigarettes. *Front. Pharmacol.* **2016**, *7*, 279. [CrossRef]

61. Phillip, J. Could CBD oil replace drug treatments for sarcoidosis? Available online: https://marijuanastocks.com/could-cbd-oil-replace-drug-treatments-for-sarcoidosis/ (accessed on 27 February 2017).

62. Cunningham, D.; Teichtahl, H.; Hunt, J.M.; Dow, C.; Valentine, R. Necrotizing pulmonary granulomata in a marijuana smoker. *Chest* **2000**, *117*, 1511–1514.

63. Madsen, L.R.; Krarup, N.; Bergmann, T.K.; Baerentzen, S.; Neghabat, S.; Duval, L.; Knudsen, S.T. A Cancer that went up in smoke: Pulmonary reaction to e-cigarettes imitating metastatic cancer. *Chest* **2016**, *149*, e65–e67. [CrossRef] [PubMed]

64. Crommelin, H.A.; Vorselaars, A.; van Moorsel, C.H.; Korenromp, I.H.; Deneer, V.H.; Grutters, J.C. Anti-TNF therapeutics for the treatment of sarcoidosis. *Immunotherapy* **2014**, *6*, 1127–1143. [CrossRef] [PubMed]

65. Baha, A.; Hanazay, C.; Kokturk, N.; Turktas, H. A Case of Sarcoidosis Associated With Anti-Tumor Necrosis Factor Treatment. *J. Investig. Med. High Impact Case Rep.* **2015**, *3*, 2324709615571366. [CrossRef] [PubMed]

66. Butnor, K.J. Pulmonary sarcoidosis induced by interferon-alpha therapy. *Am. J. Surg. Pathol.* **2005**, *29*, 976–979. [CrossRef] [PubMed]

67. Davis, K.L.; Agarwal, A.; Verma, A.R. Checkpoint inhibition in pediatric hematologic malignancies. *Pediatr. Hematol. Oncol.* **2017**, *34*, 379–394. [CrossRef]

68. Lucchesi, M.; Sardi, I.; Puppo, G.; Chella, A.; Favre, C. The dawn of "immune-revolution" in children: Early experiences with checkpoint inhibitors in childhood malignancies. *Cancer Chemother. Pharmacol.* **2017**, *80*, 1047–1053. [CrossRef]

69. Dunn-Pirio, A.M.; Shah, S.; Eckstein, C. Neurosarcoidosis following Immune Checkpoint Inhibitio. *Case Rep. Oncol.* **2018**, *11*, 521–526. [CrossRef]

70. Casanova, N.; Zhou, T.; Knox, K.S.; Garcia, J.G.N. Identifying Novel Biomarkers in Sarcoidosis Using Genome-Based Approaches. *Clin. Chest Med.* **2015**, *36*, 621–630. [CrossRef]

71. Ukae, S.; Tsutsumi, H.; Adachi, N.; Takahashi, H.; Kato, F.; Chiba, S. Preschool sarcoidosis manifesting as juvenile rheumatoid arthritis: A case report and a review of the literature of Japanese cases. *Pediatr. Int.* **1994**, *36*, 515–518. [CrossRef]

72. Teirstein, A.S.; Judson, M.; Baughman, R.P.; Rossman, M.D.; Yeager, H., Jr.; Moller, D.R.; Case Control Etiologic Study of Sarcoidosis (ACCESS) Writing Group. The spectrum of biopsy sites for the diagnosis of sarcoidosis. *Sarcoidosis Vasc. Diffus. Lung Dis.* **2005**, *22*, 139–146.

73. Hutchinson, J. *Case of Livid Papillary Psoriasis*; J&A Churchill: London, UK, 1877; Volume 1.

74. Boeck, C. Multiple benign sarcoid of the skin. *J. Cutan Genitourin. Dis.* **1899**, *17*, 543–550.

75. Moller, D.R.; Rybicki, B.; Hamzeh, N.Y.; Montgomery, C.G.; Chen, E.S.; Drake, W.; Fontenot, A.P. Genetic, Immunologic, and Environmental Basis of Sarcoidosis. *Ann. Am. Thorac. Soc.* **2017**, *14*, S429–S436. [CrossRef] [PubMed]

76. Kaiser, Y.; Lepzien, R.; Kullberg, S.; Eklund, A.; Smed-Sörensen, A.; Grunewald, J. Expanded lung T-bet+RORγT+ CD4+ T-cells in sarcoidosis patients with a favourable disease phenotype. *Eur. Respir. J.* **2016**, *48*, 484–494. [CrossRef]

77. Schupp, J.C.; Tchaptchet, S.; Lützen, N.; Engelhard, P.; Müller-Quernheim, J.; Freudenberg, M.A.; Prasse, A. Immune response to Propionibacterium acnes in patients with sarcoidosis–in vivo and in vitro. *BMC Pulm. Med.* **2015**, *15*, 75. [CrossRef]

78. Broos, C.E.; van Nimwegen, M.; Kleinjan, A.; ten Berge, B.; Muskens, F.; in 't Veen, J.C.; Annema, J.T.; Lambrecht, B.N.; Hoogsteden, H.C.; Hendriks, R.W.; et al. Impaired survival of regulatory T cells in pulmonary sarcoidosis. *Respir. Res.* **2015**, *16*, 108. [CrossRef]

79. Hetherington, S. Sarcoidosis in young children. *Am. J. Dis. Child.* **1982**, *136*, 13–15. [CrossRef]

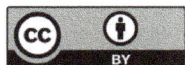

diagnostics

MDPI

Article

Left Ventricular Dysfunction and Plasmatic NT-proBNP Are Associated with Adverse Evolution in Respiratory Syncytial Virus Bronchiolitis

Moises Rodriguez-Gonzalez [1,2,*], **Alvaro Antonio Perez-Reviriego** [1,2],
Ana Castellano-Martinez [2,3], **Simon Lubian-Lopez** [2,4] **and Isabel Benavente-Fernandez** [2,4]

1   Paediatric Cardiology Division, Puerta del Mar University Hospital, 11009 Cadiz, Spain
2   Biomedical Research and Innovation Institute of Cadiz (INiBICA), Research Unit, Puerta del Mar University
     Hospital, University of Cadiz, 11009 Cadiz, Spain
3   Paediatric Nephrology Division, Puerta del Mar University Hospital, 11009 Cadiz, Spain
4   Neonatology Division, Puerta del Mar University Hospital, 11009 Cadiz, Spain
*   Correspondence: doctromoisesrodriguez@gmail.com

Received: 27 June 2019; Accepted: 26 July 2019; Published: 27 July 2019

Abstract: Aim: To investigate whether the presence of left ventricular myocardial dysfunction (LVMD) assessed by Tei index (LVTX) impacts the outcomes of healthy infants with Respiratory Syncytial Virus Bronchiolitis (RSVB). To explore whether N-terminal pro-B-type natriuretic peptide (NT-proBNP) increases the accuracy of traditional clinical markers in predicting the outcomes. Methods: A single-centre, prospective, cohort study including healthy infants aged 1–12 months old admitted for RSVB between 1 October 2016 and 1 April 2017. All patients underwent clinical, laboratory and echocardiographic evaluation within 24 h of admission. Paediatric intensive care unit (PICU) admission was defined as severe disease. Results: We enrolled 50 cases of RSVB (median age of 2 (1–6.5) months; 40% female) and 50 age-matched controls. We observed higher values of LVTX in infants with RSVB than in controls (0.42 vs. 0.36; $p = 0.008$). Up to nine (18%) children presented with LVMD (LVTX > 0.5), with a higher incidence of PICU admission (89% vs. 5%; $p < 0.001$). The diagnostic performance of NT-proBNP in predicting LVMD was high (area under the receiver operator characteristic curve (AUC) 0.95, CI 95% 0.90–1). The diagnostic yield of the predictive model for PICU admission that included NT-proBNP was excellent (AUC 0.945, CI 95% 0.880–1), and significantly higher than the model without NT-proBNP ($p = 0.026$). Conclusions: LVMD could be present in healthy infants with RSVB who develop severe disease. NT-proBNP seems to improve traditional clinical markers for outcomes.

Keywords: respiratory syncytial virus; NT-proBNP; echocardiography; pulmonary hypertension; myocardial dysfunction; tissue doppler imaging; Tei index; biomarkers; infants

1. Introduction

Respiratory Syncytial Virus Bronchiolitis (RSVB) is the leading cause of lower respiratory infection and hospital admission among children up to 2 years of age worldwide [1]. Approximately 2–6% cases of RSVB will develop a severe form of the disease, requiring admission to the paediatric intensive care unit (PICU) and mechanical ventilation (MV) [1,2]. RSVB constitutes approximately 13% of all PICU admissions [2]. Current guidelines recognize the identification of specific risk factors (congenital heart disease (CHD), chronic lung disease (CLD), prematurity, etc.) and clinical evaluation as the best tools to assess severity, predict evolution and tailor management [3].

Cardiovascular involvement seems to be a relevant prognostic factor in RSVB. Cardiovascular complications are present in up to 9% of cases of RSVB and constitute the second most common extrapulmonary manifestation after infectious complications [4]. These events usually present in an abrupt and unexpected manner in children with severe RSVB, and infants with CHD are particularly susceptible to these complications and adverse outcomes [5]. Interestingly, nearly half of the children admitted to PICU with RSVB are healthy prior to the clinical event [2]. In these patients, the presence of acute lung injury secondary to RSVB can also lead to important cardiovascular effects, especially elevated pulmonary vascular resistance and overload on the right ventricle (RV) [6–8]. Moreover, previous studies assessing the plasma levels of cardiac troponin in RSVB suggest an underrecognized yet clinically significant incidence of myocardial damage in this population [9–11]. Furthermore, RV global dysfunction in ventilated healthy infants has been reported [12]. Recently, we found that mild to moderate forms of pulmonary hypertension (PH) could impact the outcome of healthy infants with RSVB [13].

Adverse RV–LV interactions and left ventricle (LV) myocardial dysfunction (LVMD) are emerging as important determinants of PH outcomes. PH can induce complex changes in LV geometry and causes an abnormal relaxation and non-uniform contraction pattern in the LV wall, leading to LVMD [14–16]. However, most studies in healthy infants with RSVB found no abnormalities when assessing LVMD through conventional echocardiographic parameters [12,13,17–19]. Remarkably, there are no studies to date assessing LVMD in RSVB by more sensitive methods such as tissue Doppler imaging (TDI) echocardiography.

N-terminal pro-B-type natriuretic peptide (NT-proBNP) is a hormone synthesized and released into the circulation by ventricular myocytes in response to pressure/volume overload and an increase in myocardial wall stress [20]. Elevated serum NT-proBNP levels have been defined as a powerful biomarker in the diagnosis of PH, and both LVMD and RV myocardial dysfunction (RVMD) secondary to pulmonary diseases [21–25]. Of note, we recently showed how NT-proBNP could be considered an adequate biomarker for PH in previously healthy infants with RSVB [13].

In this study, we aimed to investigate the presence of adverse RV–LV interactions and LVMD (assessed by TDI-echocardiography) in previously healthy infants with RSVB. We hypothesized that acute PH with RV pressure overload may indeed have a direct impact on LV performance. We also hypothesized that those infants with LVMD are prone to developing a more severe form of disease. Finally, we sought to test NT-proBNP as a biomarker for LVMD and explore whether NT-proBNP increases the accuracy of traditional clinical markers in predicting the severity of the disease.

2. Materials and Methods

2.1. Design, Settings and Study Population

This was a single-centre, prospective, cohort study including infants aged 1–12 months old admitted to the paediatric department in our institution (a tertiary university-affiliated hospital in Spain) due to RSVB (determined by a confirmed Respiratory Syncytial Virus (RSV) antigen test) between 1 October 2016 and 1 April 2017. All patients underwent clinical, laboratory and echocardiographic evaluation within 24 h of admission. We excluded patients with co-existing CHD or CLD, prematurity, those that received MV or intravenous fluid before assessment, and those with poor-quality echocardiographic images or incomplete medical records. Severe cases were screened for coinfection and, if present, were also excluded. The control group consisted of age-matched healthy infants who underwent evaluation for heart murmur at our paediatric cardiology outpatient clinic during the study period. These controls followed the same echocardiographic protocol as study patients. Our Institutional Review Board approved the study. Informed consent was obtained for all patients.

2.2. Clinical and Laboratory Assessment and Outcomes

The bronchiolitis score of Sant Joan de Déu (BROSJOD) [26] was used to assess severity at admission clinically. A BROSJOD score greater than 10 points is indicative of a severe clinical state. Venous pH and pCO2 were determined and respiratory acidosis (RA) was diagnosed when pH

< 7.35 and pCO2 > 45 mmHg. Plasma NT-proBNP levels at admission were determined using a commercially available electrochemiluminescent immunoassay kit (ElecSys 2010, Roche Diagnostics). The primary outcome was PICU admission during hospitalization. PICU admission criteria for RSVB at our institution include the presence of: apnea, extreme bradycardia, the need for respiratory support greater than high-flow nasal cannula oxygen therapy or inotropic support.

2.3. Echocardiographic Assessment

Standard techniques to obtain M-mode, two-dimensional and Doppler (color, pulsed, continuous and TDI) echocardiograms were performed by the same experienced paediatric cardiologist (RGM) as recommended in the guidelines for the paediatric echocardiogram [27]. Images were obtained using a Phillips IE33 ultrasound scanner with an 8 or 12-MHz sectorial transducer. Each examination was recorded, and all the studies were reviewed off-line by 2 observers (RGM and PRA), who were blinded to the patient's clinical profile. All echocardiographic measurements represent the average of 3 beats. Control and case echocardiographic data were deidentified before data analysis. Figures 1 and 2 show the main echocardiographic measures used in this study.

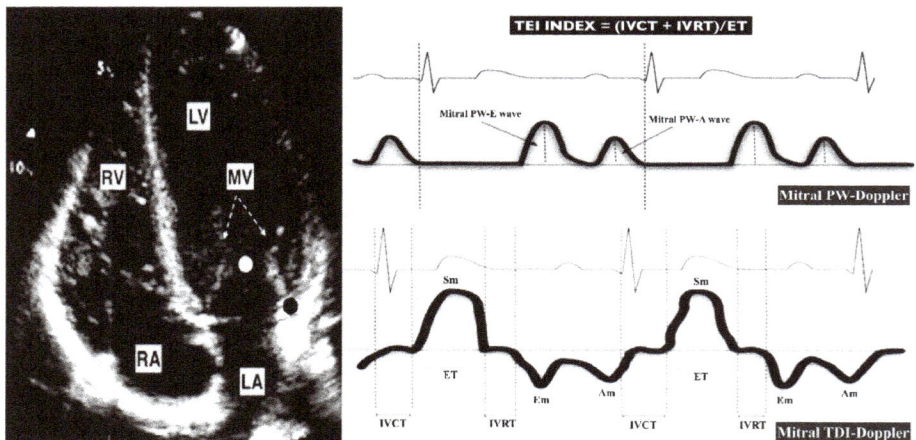

Figure 1. Echocardiographic parameters used for the estimation of LV performance. The left panel shows a four-chamber apical view. The right panel shows the waves used to assess LV performance. The Mitral PW-Doppler wave is obtained at the level of the LV inflow (white point). The Mitral TDI-Doppler wave is obtained at the level of the lateral mitral annulus (black point). MV (mitral valve; dotted arrow). RV (right ventricle). LV (left ventricle). RA (right atria). LA (left atria). PW (pulsed wave). DTI (Doppler tissue imaging). Sm (Doppler imaging (TDI)-derived peak systolic annular velocity). Em (TDI-derived early diastolic mitral annulus velocity). Am (TDI-derived late diastolic mitral annulus velocity). PW-E (PW-derived mitral peak early diastolic velocity). PW-A (PW-derived mitral peak late diastolic velocity). IVCT (TDI-derived isovolumic contraction time). IVRT (TDI-derived isovolumic relaxation time). ET (TDI-derived ejection time).

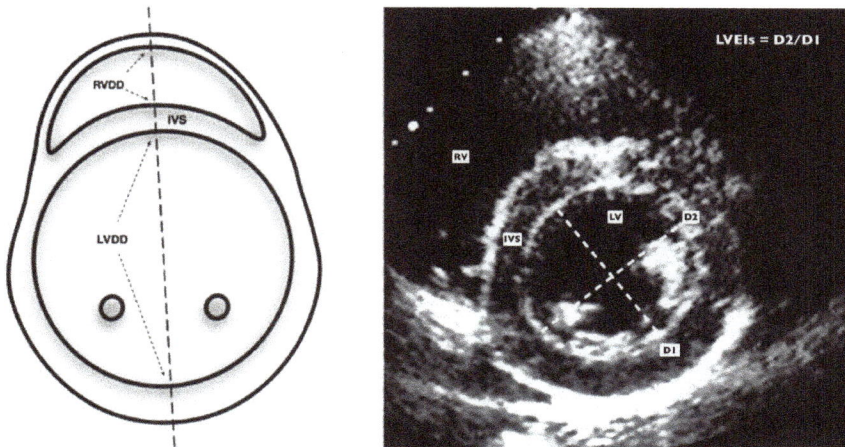

Figure 2. Echocardiographic parameters used for the estimation of RV and pulmonary hemodynamics. The figure shows a parasternal short axis view at the level of the papillary muscles. The left panel shows a schematic representation and the right panel shows real echocardiographic imaging. The LV systolic eccentricity index (LVEI) is obtained with de D2/D1 (dotted lines) ratio measured in systole as showed in the illustration. A LVEI > 1.2 is suggestive of raised RV pressures or pulmonary hypertension in infants[32]. RVDD (right ventricular diastolic diameter; dotted arrows). LVDD (left ventricular diastolic diameter; dotted arrows). IVS (Interventricular septum). RV (right ventricle). LV (left ventricle). D2 (LV systolic anteroposterior diameter). D1 (LV systolic laterolateral diameter).

2.3.1. Right-Sided Echocardiographic Assessment

The RV end-diastolic diameter (RVEDD) and the RV/LV ratio (RVLVr) were used as indicators of RV dilation. RV systolic function was assessed by the tricuspid annular plane systolic excursion (TAPSE) [28], and by the tissue Doppler imaging (TDI) derived peak systolic annular velocity at the tricuspid level of the RV free wall (St). RV Tei index (RVTX) was used as a measurement of global (systolic and diastolic) RV function. It was calculated using the TDI-derived isovolumic contraction (IVC), isovolumic relaxation (IVR) and ejection time (ET) intervals (measured at the lateral part of the tricuspid annulus) as previously described [29]. RV systolic pressure was calculated by the systolic gradient of the tricuspid regurgitation jet (TRJG) and using the simplified Bernoulli equation [30]. Due to the absence of an adequate tricuspid regurgitation jet in most patients, the RV outflow tract acceleration time/ejection time ratio (ATET) [31], the LV systolic eccentricity index (LVEI) [32], and the presence of septal flattening at the end of systole on the qualitative assessment were also used as indicators of RV systolic pressures [30]. The LVEI was also used as a measurement of leftward displacement of the interventricular septum (IVS).

2.3.2. Left-Sided Echocardiographic Assessment

The LV end-diastolic diameter (LVEDD) was used as an indicator of LV dilation. The LV shortening fraction (LVSF) and the tissue Doppler imaging (TDI)-derived peak systolic annular velocity at the mitral level of the LV free wall (Sm) were used to assess LV systolic function. To assess the diastolic LV function, we obtained the mitral peak early (E) and late (A) diastolic velocity using the pulsed wave Doppler of the mitral valve inflow. Also, the TDI-derived early diastolic mitral annulus velocity (Em) was measured at the lateral part of the mitral annulus. The E/Em ratio and E/A ratio were calculated as indicators of LV filling pressures. LV Tei index (LVTX) was used as a measurement of global (systolic and diastolic) LV function. It was calculated using the TDI-derived isovolumic contraction (IVC), isovolumic relaxation (IVR) and ejection time (ET) intervals (measured at the lateral part of the mitral annulus) as previously described [29]. Cui and Robertson reported in 2006 that the mean normal value of the LVTX for infants aged 1–12 months is 0.35 (0.09), and that a LVTX less than 0.5 is the upper limit of normal (2Zscore) [33]. Therefore, a LVTX > 0.5 was defined as LVMD in this study.

2.4. Reproductibility

To explore intra-observer and inter-observer agreement, 30 echocardiographic studies were randomly selected and analysed offline. To estimate the intra-observer agreement, the first observer (RGM) remeasured the LVTX, RVTX and LVEI with a 30-day interval blinded to previous measurements and patient information. To assess the inter-observer agreement, the means of both observers for each measurement were compared.

2.5. Statistical Analysis

Continuous data are presented as the median (range) or mean (standard deviation) after testing for normality with the Shapiro–Wilk test; categorical data are presented as frequencies and percentage. Mean comparison was performed using the Student's *t* test or Wilcoxon Mann–Whitney test as appropriate. Proportions were compared using the Chi-square test or exact methods as necessary. Pearson and Spearman coefficients were used to assess correlations between continuous data. A receiver operator curve (ROC) analysis was used to determine the diagnostic accuracy of NT-proBNP for LVMD. The best cut-off value of NT-proBNP to detect LVMD was empirically estimated based on the Liu method, and values of sensitivity (Se), specificity (Sp), negative predictive value (NPV) and positive predictive value (PPV) were calculated for the obtained cut point. We selected 2 predefined predictive models for PICU admission. The selection of the included variables was based on the theoretical background and the exploratory analysis. Model 1 (proposed model) included age, BROSJOD score and NT-proBNP levels and model 2 (traditional model) included age and BROSJOD score. Prediction models were evaluated through multivariate logistic regression analysis. The discriminating ability of each model was assessed by the area under the receiver operator characteristic (AUC) curve. The AUCs from the obtained models were then compared by using the DeLong method [34] to determine whether any model resulted in increased predictive accuracy. The reliability of echocardiographic measurements was evaluated with the intra-class correlation (ICC) coefficients and Bland–Altman (BA) analysis [35]. Based on the 95% confident interval of the ICC coefficients, values less than 0.5, between 0.5 and 0.75, between 0.75 and 0.9, and greater than 0.90 were considered indicative of poor, moderate, good, and excellent reliability, respectively. All the statistical analyses were performed using the Stata 13.0. (StataCorp. 2013. Stata Statistical Software: Release 13. College Station, TX: StataCorp LP.). A *p* value < 0.05 was considered statistically significant.

3. Results

3.1. Baseline Characteristics and Outcomes of Patients with RSVB

We enrolled a total of 50 cases of RSVB with a median age of 2 (1–6.5) months (40% female). The control group consisted of 50 healthy infants with no differences regarding age, sex or body surface area (BSA) distribution (Table 1). RSVB patients were admitted 2.76 (1.23) days after the initial symptoms, with a median BROSJOD score of 6 (1–14), a median SpO2 of 93% (87–98%), and a median heart rate of 118 bpm (89–179 bpm). Up to nine (18%) cases presented RA and a BROSJOD score > 10. A total of 10 (20%) cases needed PICU admission within 1.20 (0.38) days from hospitalization (length of PICU stay 5 (2–9) days) and were classified as having severe RSVB. A total of 3 of these 10 cases required MV and seven of them required continuous positive airway pressure (CPAP). No cases of arrhythmia different from sinus tachycardia were observed. No patient required inotropic support and none of the included patients died.

Table 1. Baseline clinical and laboratory characteristics of the Respiratory Syncytial Virus Bronchiolitis (RSVB) population and comparison with controls.

Variable	RSVB Group (*n* = 50)	Control Group (*n* = 50)	*p* Value
Age (months)	2 (1–6.5)	2 (1–9)	0.591
Female sex	20 (40)	23 (46)	0.545
BSA (m2)	0.28 (0.18–0.43)	0.27 (0.18–0.42)	0.617
Time of symptoms (days)	2.76 (1.23)	-	-
BROSJOD score	6 (1–14)	-	-
SpO2 (%)	93 (87–98)	99 (95–100)	<0.001
Heart rate (bpm)	118 (89–179)	109 (87–133)	0.002
pH	7.36 (7.22–7.45)	-	-
pCO2	42 (31–71)	-	-
Nt-proBNP (pg/mL)	511 (62–5532)	-	-
Respiratory Acidosis	9 (18)	-	-
BROSJOD > 10	9 (18)	-	-
PICU admission	10 (20)	-	-

BSA (body surface area); PICU (paediatric intensive care unit); BROSJOD score (bronchiolitis score of Sant Joan de Déu); Nt-proBNP (N-terminal pro-B-type natriuretic peptide); PICU (Paediatric intensive care unit).

3.2. Echocardiographic Alterations in Patients with RSVB

The RSVB group had a higher proportion of pericardial effusion (34% vs. 6%; *p* < 0.001). All cases of pericardial effusion were mild and did not require any treatment. We observed higher values of LVTX (0.42 vs. 0.36; *p* = 0.008) in infants with RSVB than in controls (Figure 3). The RSVB group also presented more cases of septal flattening (28% vs. 6%; *p* = 0.003), and higher TRJG (27 vs. 22 mmHg; *p* = 0.013), RVTX (0.39 vs. 0.36; *p* = 0.005) and LVEI (1.08 vs. 1; *p* < 0.001) than the control group. There were no differences between RSVB and control groups regarding echocardiographic parameters of ventricular dimensions, systolic or diastolic function (Table 2).

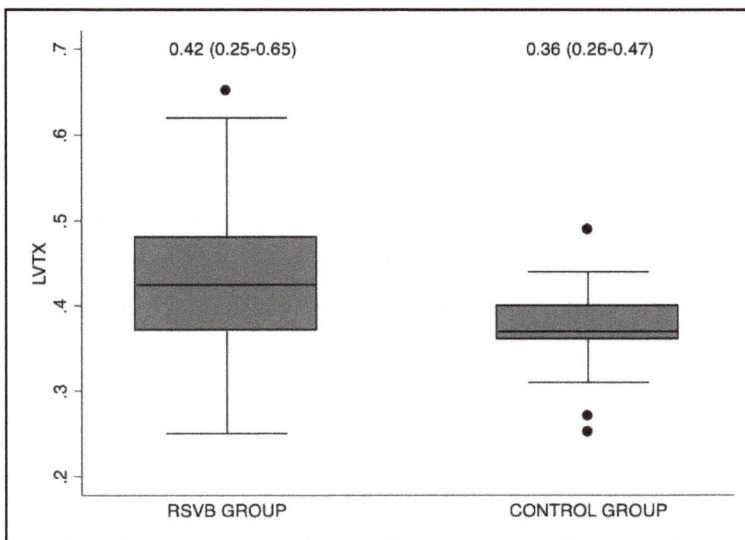

Figure 3. Box-plot diagram showing that the cases of RSVB presented higher values of LVTX at admission than healthy controls (*p* = 0.008). LVTX (Left ventricular Tei index).

Table 2. Baseline echocardiographic characteristics of the RSVB population and comparison with controls.

Variable	RSVB Group (*n* = 50)	Control Group (*n* = 50)	*p* Value
Pericardial effusion	17 (34)	3 (6)	<0.001
Left ventricle			
LVDD (mm)	21 (17–29)	21 (14–28)	0.470
LVSF (%)	38.5 (5.6)	39 (5)	0.851
Sm (cm/s)	8.7 (1.6)	9 (1.2)	0.573
Mitral E (cm/s)	98 (79–125)	96 (76–123)	0.798
Mitral A (cm/s)	75 (49–97)	71 (51–93)	0.259
Mitral E/A	1.25 (0.93–1.98)	1.43 (1–2)	0.200
Mitral Em (cm/s)	9.4 (6–5–14)	10 (6.6–15)	0.110
Mitral Am (cm/s)	9 (5–15)	9 (6–13)	0.182
Mitral E/Em (cm/s)	10.2 (5.8–20)	9.8 (5.2–17)	0.283
LVTX	0.42 (0.25–0.65)	0.36 (0.26–0.47)	0.008
Right ventricle			
RVDD (mm)	10 (7–19)	10 (7–14)	0.264
RV/LV ratio	0.49 (0.28–0.80)	0.46 (0.28–0.76)	0.473
TAPSE (mm)	12.3 (1.6)	12 (1.8)	0.624
St (cm/s)	8.5 (2)	9.1 (1.7)	0.901
RVTX	0.39 (0.25–0.65)	0.37 (0.26–0.48)	0.005
Adequate TRJ	25 (50)	30 (60)	0.633
TRJG (mmHg)	27 (18–47)	22 (16–34)	0.013
ATET	0.38 (0.06)	0.39 (0.03)	0.288
LVEI	1.08 (0.98–1.45)	1 (0.95–1.12)	<0.001
Septal Flattening	14 (28)	3 (6)	0.003

LVDD (left ventricle diastolic diameter); LVSF (left ventricular shortening fraction); LVTX (left ventricular Tei index); RVDD (right ventricular diastolic diameter); RV (right ventricle); LV (Left ventricle); TAPSE (tricuspid annular plane systolic excursion); RVTX (Right ventricular Tei index); TRJ (tricuspid regurgitation jet); TRJG (tricuspid regurgitation jet gradient); ATET (right ventricular acceleration time/right ventricular ejection time ratio); LVEI (systolic left ventricular eccentricity index).

3.3. Adverse LV–RV Interactions in Patients with RSVB

In the RSVB group, increased LVTX was related to echocardiographic parameters indicating higher RV dimensions (*Rho* RVDD = 0.56, *Rho* RVLVr = 0.60), higher RV pressures (*Rho* TRJG = 0.54, *Rho* ATET = −0.50, *Rho* LVEI = 0.77), and decreased RV global function (*Rho* RVTX= 0.74). We did not find associations of echocardiographic measurements of RV systolic function (TAPSE and St) with LVTX (Table 3 and Figure 4).

Table 3. Correlation coefficients between LVTX and RV echocardiographic parameters and plasmatic NT-proBNP levels in RSVB cases.

Variable	Rho	*p* Value
RVDD	0.56	0.003
RV/LV ratio	0.60	0.001
TAPSE	−0.19	0.159
St	−0.12	0.217
RVTX	0.738	<0.001
TRJG	0.54	0.004
ATET	−0.50	0.009
LVEI	0.77	<0.001
NT-proBNP	0.73	<0.001

RVDD (right ventricular diastolic diameter); RV (right ventricle); LV (Left ventricle); TAPSE (tricuspid annular plane systolic excursion); RVTX (Right ventricular Tei index); TRJ (tricuspid regurgitation jet); TRJG (tricuspid regurgitation jet gradient); ATET (right ventricular acceleration time/right ventricular ejection time ratio); LVEI (systolic left ventricular eccentricity index).

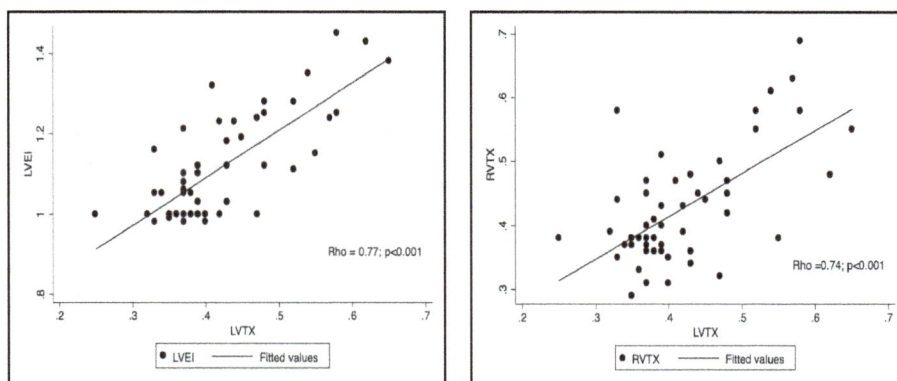

Figure 4. A representation of the correlation found between LVTX and parameters of RV function (RVTX, right panel) and RV pressures (LVEI, left panel). LVTX (Left ventricular Tei index). RVTX (right ventricular Tei index). LVEI (systolic left ventricular eccentricity index).

3.4. LVMD in Patients with RSVB

We found LVMD, defined by a LVTX > 0.5, in nine (18%) patients with RSVB (Table 4). LVMD was associated with PICU admission (89% vs. 5%; $p < 0.001$). These patients presented with a higher BROSJOD score (11 vs. 6; $p < 0.001$), lower SpO2 (90% vs. 94%; $p < 0.001$), more cases of RA (55% vs. 9%; $p = 0.001$), and higher NT-proBNP levels (2221 pg/mL vs. 377 pg ml; $p < 0.001$) than those with a normal LV myocardial function. The LVTX was also strongly correlated with NT-proBNP levels ($Rho = 0.73$) (Figure 5).

Table 4. Clinical and laboratory characteristics in patients with RSVB and LVMD, and comparison with those patients with normal LV function.

Variable	LVMD (n = 9; 18%)	Normal LV Function (n = 41; 82%)	p Value
Age (months)	2 (1–4.5)	2 (1–6.5)	0.538
Female sex	2 (22)	18 (44)	0.230
BSA (m^2)	0.29 (0.18–0.33)	0.28 (0.18–0.43)	0.742
Time of symptoms (days)	2 (1.5)	3 (1–7)	0.488
BROSJOD score	11 (9–14)	6 (1–13)	<0.001
SpO2 (%)	90 (87–93)	94 (88–98)	<0.001
Heart rate (bpm)	135 (100–164)	116 (89–179)	0.141
pH	7.3 (7.25–7.42)	7.36 (7.22–7.45)	0.115
pCO2 (mmHg)	54 (31–61)	41 (31–71)	0.009
Nt-proBNP (pg/mL)	2221 (891–5532)	377 (62–1779)	<0.001
PICU admission	8 (89)	2 (5)	<0.001

LVMD (left ventricular myocardial dysfunction); BSA (Body surface area); PICU (paediatric intensive care unit).

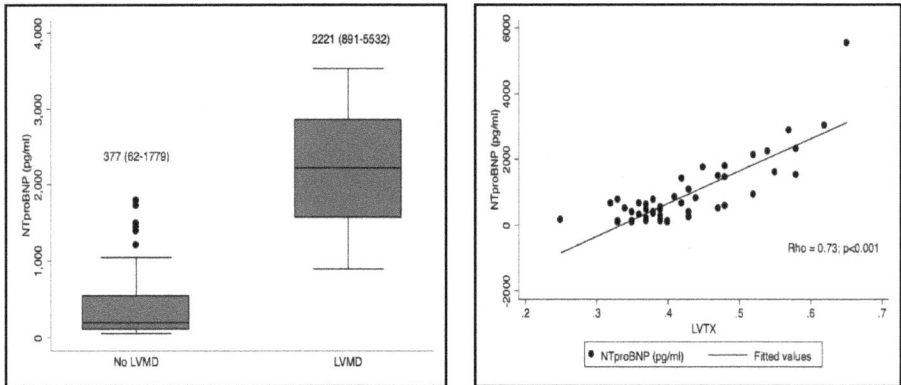

Figure 5. The left panel is a box-plot diagram representing the comparison of NT-proBNP levels between patients with and without LVMD. The right panel represents the correlation found between LVTX and NT-proBNP levels. LVTX (Left ventricular Tei index); LVMD (Left ventricular myocardial dysfunction).

3.5. NT-ProBNP as Biomarker for LVMD

The diagnostic performance of NT-proBNP to predict LVMD in infants with RSVB resulted in an area under the ROC curve of 0.91 (CI95% 0.79–0.98) (Figure 6). The best estimated cut-off value to predict LVMD on echocardiography was 1500 pg/mL, correctly classifying 92% of cases, with a Se of 0.80 (CI95% 0.49–0.94), Sp of 0.95 (CI95% 0.83–0.98), a PPV of 0.80 (CI95% 0.49–0.94), and an NPV of 0.95 (CI95% 0.87–0.99) (Youden index 0.75).

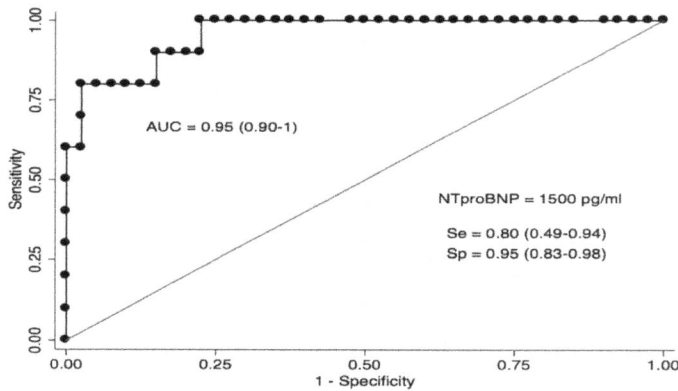

Figure 6. Representation of the receiver operating characteristic curve of NT-proBNP to detect LVMD in infants with RSVB. LVMD (Left ventricular myocardial dysfunction).

3.6. Clinical and Laboratory Predictors of PICU Admission in RSVB

We developed two different and predefined prediction models for PICU admission in RSVB. The variables used were clinical parameters that are traditionally used to assess severity in RSVB (age and clinical score), and NT-proBNP as biomarker for LVMD. Model 1 (the proposed model) included age < 3 months, BROSJOD score > 10, and NT-proBNP > 1500 pg/mL. Model 2 (the traditional model) included age < 3 months and BROSJOD score > 10. The diagnostic yield of model 1 for PICU admission was excellent (AUC 0.945, CI95% 0.880–1), and significantly higher than the yield for model 2 ($p = 0.026$). In model 1, the presence of NT-proBNP levels > 1500 pg/mL was the only independent predictive factor for PICU admission in RSVB, with an OR 27.03 (CI95% (1.50–487), *p* = 0.025) (Table 5 and Figure 7).

Table 5. Univariate and Multivariate logistic regression analysis performed to find a predictive model for PICU admission during hospitalization in our RSVB cohort.

Variable	Univariate Analysis OR (CI 95%)	*p* Value	Multivariate Analysis OR (CI 95%)	*p* Value	pseudoR2
Model 1				<0.001	0.51
Age < 3 months	0.88 (0.19–4.04)	0.875	0.71 (0.66–7.58)	0.777	
BROSJOD score > 10	44.33 (6.22–315.50)	<0.001	3.06 (0.12–76.44)	0.494	
NT-proBNP > 1500 pg/mL	76 (9.27–622)	<0.001	27.03 (1.50–487)	0.025	
Model 2				<0.001	0.38
Age < 3 months	0.88 (0.19–4.04)	0.875	0.52 (0.06–4.21)	0.541	
BROSJOD score > 10	44.33 (6.22–315.50)	<0.001	49.27 (6.38–380)	<0.001	

OR (Odds ratio); CI (Confidence interval).

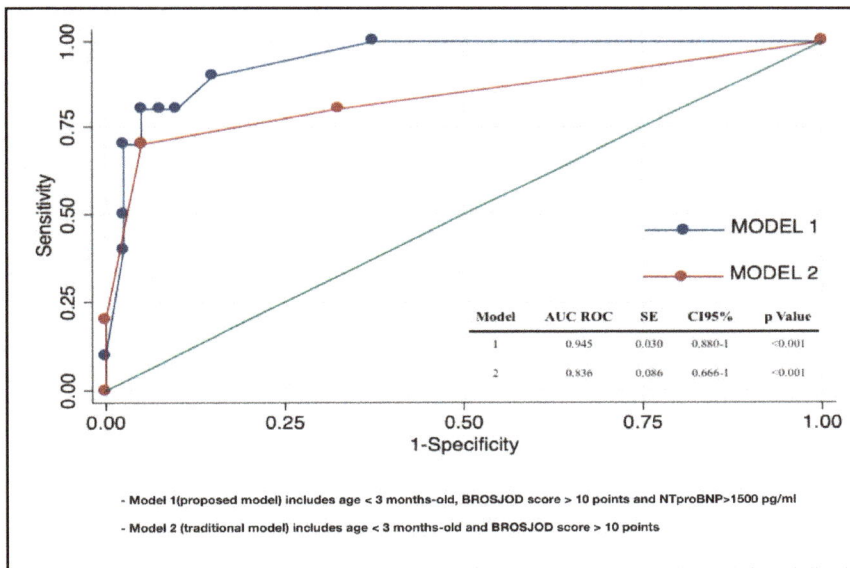

Model	AUC ROC	SE	CI95%	p Value
1	0.945	0.030	0.880-1	<0.001
2	0.836	0.086	0.666-1	<0.001

- Model 1(proposed model) includes age < 3 months-old, BROSJOD score > 10 points and NTproBNP>1500 pg/ml
- Model 2 (traditional model) includes age < 3 months-old and BROSJOD score > 10 points

Figure 7. Graphical representation of the comparison between the areas under the receiver operator characteristic curves of the predictive models selected.

3.7. Reproductibility

The intra-observer and inter-observer agreement for LVTX, RVTX and LVEI were good or excellent, with all ICC coefficients > 0.75 (Table 6).

Table 6. Intra-observer and inter-observer agreement scores for the main echocardiographic measurements performed in this study, the left ventricular and right ventricular Tei indexes (LVTX and RVTX), and the systolic left ventricular eccentricity index (LVEI).

Variable	Intra-observer (RG.M)		Inter-observer (RG.M and PR.A)	
	ICC (95% CI)	BA (LOA)	ICC (95% CI)	BA (LOA)
LVTX	0.95 (0.93–0.99)	0.00 (−0.03–0.03)	0.84 (0.74–0.93)	−0.01 (−0.07–0.05)
RVTX	0.97 (0.95–0.99)	−0.002 (−0.02–0.02)	0.86 (0.77–0.95)	−0.015 (−0.07–0.04)
LVEI	0.89 (0.82–0.96)	−0.007 (−0.04–0.03)	0.84 (0.73–0.94)	−0.01 (−0.05–0.03)

ICC (interclass coefficient); CI (confidence interval); BA (Bland–Altman average); LOA (limits of agreement).

4. Discussion

The main finding of our study is that LVMD was observed at the early stages of the disease in up to 18% of previously healthy infants with RSVB when assessed by DTI-derived LVTX. The LVMD was associated with a more severe respiratory state, PICU admission, and echocardiographic signs of RV pressure overload and RVMD, indicating the presence of adverse RV–LV interactions in cases of severe RSVB. Also, we observed that NT-proBNP accurately identified LVMD. Moreover, we found an added benefit to the addition of NT-proBNP to the clinical evaluation in predicting the development of severe disease in this population.

CHD is an important cause of morbidity and mortality in RSVB [5]. This may be related to multiple physiological factors including baseline compromised cardiorespiratory function and the potential development of PH. However, little is known about LVMD and its association with RV function, pulmonary hemodynamics, and outcomes in previously healthy infants with RSVB. In accordance with the literature, the present study reveals that conventional parameters of myocardial function are not altered in RSVB [17–19]. Only one previous study has assessed myocardial performance using the TEI index in RSVB [12]. Our results are consistent with those reported by Thorburn et al. who found RVMD in ventilated patients with severe RSVB. However, they did not demonstrate any association between PH and RVMD. This may be due to the use of TRJG alone as an echocardiographic marker of RV pressure, and the presence of PH may had been underestimated. In a recent work from our group, we used a combination of different echocardiographic parameters to assess RV pressures and PH was reported in up to 22% of RSVB cases at early stages of the disease. In agreement with Thorburn et al., we did not find an association between PH and RV or LVMD [13]. We assessed ventricular function only by conventional parameters (TAPSE and LVSF).

To the best of our knowledge, this is the first study to evaluate LVMD using TDI-derived LVTX, and to assess RV–LV interactions in infants with RSVB. LVTX, which includes both systolic and diastolic time intervals to assess the global cardiac dysfunction, is an easily performable, recordable and reproducible parameter with normal reference values that can be applied to the entire spectrum of the paediatric population, regardless of age, heart rate, and BSA [36]. Using LVTX, we found LVMD in nearly 20% of cases. The RV shares muscle fibres, the inter-ventricular septum (IVS), and the pericardial sac with the LV. Consequently, changes in RV affect the LV, a concept termed ventricular interdependence [16,37,38]. In this study, we observed a moderate to strong correlation between LVTX and leftward displacement of the IVS (LVEI), raised RV pressures (TRGJ, ATET) and reduced RV global function (RVTX), confirming the presence of adverse RV–LV interactions in cases with severe RSVB. These results do not imply casualty, but in the absence of primary (myocarditis, cardiomyopathies, CHD) or secondary (sepsis, severe acidosis...) causes of LVMD, we suggest RV pressure overload and RV dysfunction due to pulmonary disease as the underlying condition for LVMD in our RSVB cohort. Recent paediatric studies have reported that PH can induce complex changes in LV geometry and causes an abnormal relaxation and non-uniform contraction pattern in the LV wall, leading to LVMD [14–16], supporting our hypothesis. These observations could add new insights into the pathophysiology of RSVB, highlighting a key role of the cardiovascular system, especially LV myocardial performance in this setting. Validating our findings in similar populations in different settings may also provide a basis to implement new therapeutic approaches for this disease, which currently has no effective treatment. Possible new therapeutic approaches may include the initiation of early respiratory support in cases with increased NT-proBNP, pulmonary vasodilators to reduce RV pressure overload and avoiding epinephrine in cases with LVMD.

In RSVB, the major goals are the prevention and early identification of infants at risk for severe disease in order to provide the best management options and decrease morbidity. Current guidelines recommend only clinical observation for this purpose in infants without known comorbidities [3]. However, most clinical scores for RSVB are not well validated and fail to predict outcomes [39,40]. Recently, the BROSJOD score, a validated clinical score for RSVB, has shown a strong capacity to predict the evolution in the course of RSVB, but it is not yet generalizable due to the single-centre character of the study [26]. In this context, the identification of novel biomarkers with adequate predictive value for disease severity in RSVB is an area of increasing research interest. Neutrophins, cytokines and leukotrienes are promising but not widely available for clinical practice [41]. Previous studies have also tested cardiac troponin as a prognostic marker with inconsistent results [9,10,12,13]. The LVMD found in our population was only identifiable by TDI-echocardiography, suggesting that it was mild in most of our patients. Nevertheless, this does not mean that LVMD is inconsequential in RSVB. Remarkably, most patients with LVMD presented with severe disease at admission and most of them required PICU admission. Of note, we included non-ventilated infants at early stages of the disease (mean time of 2.76 (1.23) days after the initial symptoms), when the patients had not yet been admitted to the PICU, increasing the prognostic value of our results. Therefore, assessing and understanding myocardial function in RSVB seems to be relevant.

Another interesting finding of our study was that NT-proBNP could be a useful biomarker for LVMD and subsequent outcomes in RSVB. Previous studies have also documented the correlation between LVTX and NT-proBNP plasma levels [42–44]. We explored the diagnostic accuracy of NT-proBNP to detect LVTX > 0.50, which was high (AUC 0.91), with an optimal cut-off value of 1500 pg/mL (Se 0.80, Sp 0.95, PPV 0.80, NPV 0.95). We also tested the benefit in adding NT-proBNP to the currently used clinical data to assess outcomes in RSVB. Although the predictive models including age and BROSJOD score presented a high predictive accuracy for PICU admission in our population, we observed that the addition of NT-proBNP to this model increased the predictive value significantly, and that NT-proBNP was the only independent factor within the analysed values that predicted a severe course of the disease. Most cases of RSVB are mild forms manageable on an outpatient basis without the need for laboratory exams. Nevertheless, many children sufficiently ill to require hospitalization will routinely have laboratory studies drawn. Adding NT-proBNP measurement to these studies could be useful in order to identify high-risk patients who benefit from echocardiographic screening to PH, RVMD or LVMD. Based on our results, it might be reasonable to perform an echocardiogram in those patients with NT-proBNP levels > 1500 pg/mL.

This work included some limitations. Our study was performed at a single centre and with a relatively small size. We excluded irritable or unstable patients, where the technical difficulties due to respiratory comorbidity and the patient's inability to tolerate the evaluation could impact the results. The PICU admission criteria and, subsequently, the definition of severe diseases in the study are based on the protocol of our hospital, which can vary between institutions. Therefore, a larger multicentre cohort study including irritable or unstable cases and with uniform PICU admission criteria may be needed for the verification and generalization of our results. Finally, the assessment of myocardial function and PH on echocardiography was not confirmed by an independent gold-standard method, such as cardiac magnetic resonance imaging or right heart catheterization, and therefore some patients could have been misclassified.

5. Conclusions

Adverse RV–LV interactions and LVMD could be present in healthy infants with RSVB during the early stages of the disease, negatively impacting the outcome. NT-proBNP seems to be an adequate biomarker for LVMD. Adding NT-proBNP to traditional clinical markers to assess outcomes in RSVB could improve the early detection of those cases that will develop a severe illness. Future research is need in order to confirm these results and to design new therapeutic approaches based on them.

Author Contributions: Conceptualization, M.R.-G.; methodology, M.R.-G. and I.B.-F.; software, M.R.-G. and I.B.-F.; validation, M.R.-G., I.B.-F., A.A.P.-R., A.C.-M., S.L.-L.; formal analysis, M.R.-G. and I.B.-F.; investigation, M.R.-G., A.A.P.-R. and A.C.-M.; resources, M.R.-G. and S.L.-L.; data curation, M.R.-G., A.C.-M. and A.A.P.-R.; writing—original draft preparation, M.R.-G.; writing—review and editing, M.R.-G., I.B.-F., A.A.P.-R., A.C.-M., S.L.-L.; visualization, M.R.-G. and I.B.-F.; supervision, M.R.-G. and I.B.-F.; project administration, M.R.-G.

Funding: This research received no external funding.

Conflicts of Interest: The authors declare no conflict of interest.

References

1. Hasegawa, K.; Tsugawa, Y.; Brown, D.F.M.; Mansbach, J.M.; Camargo, C.A. Trends in bronchiolitis hospitalizations in the United States, 2000–2009. Pediatrics. *Am. Acad. Pediatr.* **2013**, *132*, 28–36.
2. Ghazaly, M.; Nadel, S. Characteristics of children admitted to intensive care with acute bronchiolitis. *Eur. J. Pediatr.* **2018**, *177*, 913–920. [CrossRef] [PubMed]
3. Ralston, S.L.; Lieberthal, A.S.; Meissner, H.C.; Alverson, B.K.; Baley, J.E.; Gadomski, A.M.; Johnson, D.W.; Light, M.J.; Maraga, N.F.; Mendonca, E.A.; et al. Clinical practice guideline: The diagnosis, management, and prevention of bronchiolitis. *Am. Acad. Pediatr.* **2014**, *134*, e1474–e1502. [CrossRef] [PubMed]
4. Willson, D.F.; Landrigan, C.P.; Horn, S.D.; Smout, R.J. Complications in infants hospitalized for bronchiolitis or respiratory syncytial virus pneumonia. *J. Pediatr.* **2003**, *143*, S142–S149. [CrossRef]
5. Tulloh, R.M.; Medrano-Lopez, C.; Checchia, P.A.; Stapper, C.; Sumitomo, N.; Gorenflo, M.; Bae, E.J.; Juanico, A.; Gil-Jaurena, J.M.; Wu, M.H.; et al. CHD and respiratory syncytial virus: Global expert exchange recommendations. *Cardiol. Young* **2017**, *27*, 1504–1521. [CrossRef] [PubMed]
6. Fitzgerald, D.; Davis, G.M.; Rohlicek, C.; Gottesman, R. Quantifying pulmonary hypertension in ventilated infants with bronchiolitis: A pilot study. *J. Paediatr. Child Health* **2001**, *37*, 64–66. [CrossRef] [PubMed]
7. Bardi-Peti, L.; Ciofu, E.P. Bronchiolitis and pulmonary hypertension. *Pneumologia* **2010**, *59*, 95–100. [PubMed]
8. Kimura, D.; McNamara, I.F.; Wang, J.; Fowke, J.H.; West, A.N.; Philip, R. Pulmonary hypertension during respiratory syncytial virus bronchiolitis: A risk factor for severity of illness. *Cardiol. Young* **2019**, *20*, 1–5. [CrossRef] [PubMed]
9. Clark, S.J.; Eisenhut, M.; Sidaras, D.; Hancock, S.W.; Newland, P.; Thorburn, K. Myocardial injury in infants ventilated on the paediatric intensive care unit: A case control study. *Crit. Care* **2006**, *10*, R128. [CrossRef]
10. Moynihan, J.A.; Brown, L.; Sehra, R.; Checchia, P.A. Cardiac troponin I as a predictor of respiratory failure in children hospitalized with respiratory syncytial virus (RSV) infections: A pilot study. *Am. J. Emerg. Med.* **2003**, *21*, 479–482. [CrossRef]
11. Thorburn, K. Cardiac Troponin T levels and myocardial involvement in children with severe respiratory syncytial virus lung disease. *Acta Paediatr.* **2004**, *93*, 887–890.
12. Thorburn, K.; Eisenhut, M.; Shauq, A.; Narayanswamy, S.; Burgess, M. Right ventricular function in children with severe respiratory syncytial virus (RSV) bronchiolitis. *Minerva Anestesiol.* **2011**, *77*, 46–53. [PubMed]
13. Rodriguez-Gonzalez, M.; Benavente Fernández, I.; Castellano-Martinez, A.; Lechuga-Sancho, A.M.; Lubián-López, S.P. NT-proBNP plasma levels as biomarkers for pulmonary hypertension in healthy infants with respiratory syncytial virus infection. *Biomark. Med.* **2019**, *3*. [CrossRef] [PubMed]
14. Driessen, M.M.P.; Meijboom, F.J. Adverse ventricular-ventricular interactions in right ventricular pressure load: Insights from pediatric pulmonary hypertension versus pulmonary stenosis. *Physiol. Rep.* **2016**, *4*, e12833. [CrossRef] [PubMed]
15. Burkett, D.A.; Slorach, C.; Patel, S.S.; Redington, A.N.; Ivy, D.D.; Mertens, L.; Younoszai, A.K.; Friendberg, M.K. Impact of Pulmonary Hemodynamics and Ventricular Interdependence on Left Ventricular Diastolic Function in Children with Pulmonary Hypertension. *Circ. Cardiovasc. Imaging* **2016**, *9*, e004612. [CrossRef] [PubMed]

16. Motoji, Y.; Tanaka, H.; Fukuda, Y.; Sano, H.; Ryo, K.; Imanishi, J.; Miyoshi, T.; Sawa, T.; Mochizuki, Y.; Matsumoto, K.; et al. Interdependence of right ventricular systolic function and left ventricular filling and its association with outcome for patients with pulmonary hypertension. *Int. J. Cardiovasc. Imaging* **2015**, *23*, 691–698. [CrossRef]

17. Pahl, E.; Gidding, S.S. Echocardiographic assessment of cardiac function during respiratory syncytial virus infection. *Pediatrics* **1988**, *81*, 830–834. [PubMed]

18. Esposito, S.; Salice, P.; Bosis, S.; Ghiglia, S.; Tremolati, E.; Tagliabue, C.; Gualtieri, L.; Barbier, P.; Galeone, C.; Marchisio, P.; et al. Altered cardiac rhythm in infants with bronchiolitis and respiratory syncytial virus infection. *BMC Infect Dis.* **2010**, *24*, 305. [CrossRef]

19. Horter, T.; Nakstad, B.; Ashtari, O.; Solevåg, A.L. Right and left ventricular function in hospitalized children with respiratory syncytial virus infection. *Infect. Drug Resist.* **2017**, *10*, 419–424. [CrossRef]

20. Martinez-Rumayor, A.; Richards, A.M.; Burnett, J.C.; Januzzi, J.L., Jr. Biology of the Natriuretic Peptides. *Am. J. Cardiol.* **2008**, *101*, S3–S8. [CrossRef]

21. Kate ten, C.A.; Tibboel, D.; Kraemer, U.S. B-type natriuretic peptide as a parameter for pulmonary hypertension in children. A systematic review. *Eur. J. Pediatr.* **2015**, *23*, 1267–1275. [CrossRef] [PubMed]

22. Takatsuki, S.; Wagner, B.D.; Ivy, D.D. B-type natriuretic peptide and amino-terminal pro-B-type natriuretic peptide in pediatric patients with pulmonary arterial hypertension. *Congenit Heart Dis.* **2012**, *7*, 259–267. [CrossRef] [PubMed]

23. Hauser, J.A.; Demyanets, S.; Rusai, K.; Goritschan, C.; Weber, M.; Panesar, D.; Rindler, L.; Taylor, A.M.; Marculescus, R.; Burch, M.; et al. Diagnostic performance and reference values of novel biomarkers of paediatric heart failure. *Heart* **2016**, *27*, 1633–1639. [CrossRef] [PubMed]

24. Mladosievicova, B.; Urbanova, D.; Radvanska, E.; Slavkovsky, P.; Simkova, I. Role of NT-proBNP in detection of myocardial damage in childhood leukemia survivors treated with and without anthracyclines. *J. Exp. Clin. Cancer Res.* **2012**, *11*, 1. [CrossRef] [PubMed]

25. Li, Q.; Cui, C.-Y.; Zhang, C.; Guo, S.-Y.; Zhang, Q. On the changes of NT-proBNP level in children having undergone radical operation of tetralogy of Fallot and the clinical significance. *Eur. Rev. Med. Pharmacol. Sci.* **2015**, *19*, 3018–3022. [PubMed]

26. Balaguer, M.; Alejandre, C.; Vila, D.; Esteban, E.; Carrasco, J.L.; Cambra, F.J.; Jordan, I. Bronchiolitis Score of Sant Joan de Déu: BROSJOD Score, validation and usefulness. *Pediatr. Pulmonol.* **2017**, *52*, 533–539. [CrossRef] [PubMed]

27. Lai, W.W.; Geva, T.; Shirali, G.S.; Frommelt, P.C.; Humes, R.A.; Brook, M.M.; Pignatelli, R.H.; Rychik, J. Guidelines and Standards for Performance of a Pediatric Echocardiogram: A Report from the Task Force of the Pediatric Council of the American Society of Echocardiography. *J. Am. Soc. Echocardiogr.* **2006**, *19*, 1413–1430. [CrossRef] [PubMed]

28. Koestenberger, M.; Ravekes, W.; Everett, A.D.; Stueger, H.P.; Heinzl, B.; Gamillscheg, A.; Cvirn, G.; Boysen, A.; Fandl, A.; Nagel, B. Right ventricular function in infants, children and adolescents: Reference values of the tricuspid annular plane systolic excursion (TAPSE) in 640 healthy patients and calculation of z score values. *J. Am. Soc. Echocardiogr.* **2009**, *22*, 715–719. [CrossRef] [PubMed]

29. Tei, C.; Dujardin, K.S.; Hodge, D.O.; Bailey, K.R.; McGoon, M.D.; Tajik, A.J.; Seward, S.B. Doppler echocardiographic index for assessment of global right ventricular function. *J. Am. Soc. Echocardiogr.* **1996**, *9*, 838–847. [CrossRef]

30. Koestenberger, M.; Apitz, C.; Abdul-Khaliq, H.; Hansmann, G. Transthoracic echocardiography for the evaluation of children and adolescents with suspected or confirmed pulmonary hypertension. Expert consensus statement on the diagnosis and treatment of paediatric pulmonary hypertension. The European Paediatric Pulmonary Vascular Disease Network, endorsed by ISHLT and D6PK. *Heart* **2016**, *102*, ii14–ii22. [PubMed]

31. Habash, S.; Laser, K.T.; Moosmann, J.; Reif, R.; Adler, W.; Glöckler, M.; Kececioglu, D.; Dittrich, S. Normal values of the pulmonary artery acceleration time (PAAT) and the right ventricular ejection time (RVET) in children and adolescents and the impact of the PAAT/RVET-index in the assessment of pulmonary hypertension. *Int. J. Cardiovasc. Imaging* **2019**, *35*, 295–306. [CrossRef] [PubMed]

32. Abraham, S.; Weismann, C.G. Left Ventricular End-Systolic Eccentricity Index for Assessment of Pulmonary Hypertension in Infants. *Echocardiography* **2016**, *16*, 910–915. [CrossRef] [PubMed]

33. Cui, W.; Roberson, D.A. Left ventricular Tei index in children: Comparison of tissue Doppler imaging, pulsed wave Doppler, and M-mode echocardiography normal values. *J. Am. Soc. Echocardiogr.* **2006**, *19*, 1438–1445. [CrossRef] [PubMed]

34. DeLong, E.R.; DeLong, D.M.; Clarke-Pearson, D.L. Comparing the areas under two or more correlated receiver operating characteristic curves: A nonparametric approach. *Biometrics* **1988**, *44*, 837–845. [CrossRef] [PubMed]

35. Koo, T.K.; Li, M.Y. A Guideline of Selecting and Reporting Intraclass Correlation Coefficients for Reliability. *Res. J. Chiropr. Med.* **2016**, *15*, 155–163. [CrossRef] [PubMed]

36. Cui, W.; Roberson, D.A.; Chen, Z.; Madronero, L.F.; Cuneo, B.F. Systolic and diastolic time intervals measured from Doppler tissue imaging: Normal values and Z-score tables, and effects of age, heart rate, and body surface area. *J. Am. Soc. Echocardiogr.* **2008**, *21*, 361–370. [CrossRef] [PubMed]

37. Burkett, D.A.; Slorach, C.; Patel, S.S.; Redington, A.N.; Ivy, D.D.; Mertens, L.; Younoszai, A.K.; Friendberg, M.K. Left Ventricular Myocardial Function in Children with Pulmonary Hypertension: Relation to Right Ventricular Performance and Hemodynamics. *Circ. Cardiovasc. Imaging* **2015**, *8*, e003260. [CrossRef]

38. Haeck, M.L.A.; Höke, U.; Marsan, N.A.; Holman, E.R.; Wolterbeek, R.; Bax, J.J.; Schalij, M.J.; Vliegen, H.W.; Delgado, V. Impact of right ventricular dyssynchrony on left ventricular performance in patients with pulmonary hypertension. *Int. J. Cardiovasc. Imaging* **2014**, *30*, 713–720. [CrossRef]

39. Bekhof, J.; Reimink, R.; Brand, P.L.P. Systematic review: Insufficient validation of clinical scores for the assessment of acute dyspnoea in wheezing children. *Paediatric. Respiratory Rev.* **2014**, *15*, 98–112. [CrossRef]

40. Destino, L.; Weisgerber, M.C.; Soung, P.; Bakalarski, D.; Yan, K.; Rehborg, R.; Wagner, D.R.; Gorelick, M.H.; Simpson, P. Validity of respiratory scores in bronchiolitis. *Hosp. Pediatr.* **2012**, *2*, 202–209. [CrossRef]

41. Brown, P.M.; Schneeberger, D.L.; Piedimonte, G. Biomarkers of respiratory syncytial virus (RSV) infection: Specific neutrophil and cytokine levels provide increased accuracy in predicting disease severity. *Paediatric. Respiratory Rev.* **2015**, *16*, 232–240. [CrossRef] [PubMed]

42. Takeuchi, D.; Saji, T.; Takatsuki, S.; Fujiwara, M. Abnormal tissue doppler images are associated with elevated plasma brain natriuretic peptide and increased oxidative stress in acute Kawasaki disease. *Circ. J.* **2007**, *71*, 357–362. [CrossRef] [PubMed]

43. Ozde, C.; Dogru, M.; Ozde, Ş.; Kayapinar, O.; Kaya, A.; Korkmaz, A. Subclinical right ventricular dysfunction in intermittent and persistent mildly asthmatic children on tissue Doppler echocardiography and serum NT-proBNP: Observational study. *Pediatr. Int.* **2018**, *60*, 1024–1032. [CrossRef] [PubMed]

44. Mikkelsen, K.V.; Møller, J.E.; Bie, P.; Ryde, H.; Videbaek, L.; Haghfelt, T. Tei index and neurohormonal activation in patients with incident heart failure: Serial changes and prognostic value. *Eur. J. Heart Failure* **2006**, *8*, 599–608. [CrossRef] [PubMed]

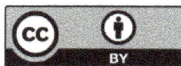

Case Report

Subcutaneous and Mediastinal Emphysema Followed by Group A Beta-Hemolytic Streptococci Mediastinitis. A Complicated Course after Adenotonsillectomy: Case Report

Anne Duvekot [1],*, Gwen van Heesch [2] and Laura Veder [1]

[1] Department of Otorhinolaryngology and head and neck surgery, Erasmus Medical Center, Sophia Children's Hospital, 3015 GD Rotterdam, The Netherlands; l.veder@erasmusmc.nl

[2] Department of Pediatrics, Pediatric Intensive Care Unit, Erasmus Medical Center, Sophia Children's Hospital, 3015 GD Rotterdam, The Netherlands; g.vanheesch@erasmusmc.nl

* Correspondence: a.duvekot@erasmusmc.nl; Tel.: +31-619-019-719

Received: 11 November 2018; Accepted: 4 December 2018; Published: 15 January 2019

Abstract: Tonsillectomy is a commonly performed surgery in the daily practice of an otorhinolaryngologist. For patients as well as health professionals, the best known complication is post-operative bleeding. Among the less noted, but potentially life-threatening, complications are the development of subcutaneous emphysema and the presence of bacteremia due to group A hemolytic streptococci. In this report, we describe a severely complicated clinical course after an uncomplicated adenotonsillectomy in a young boy. Increased awareness of relatively unknown complications after adenotonsillectomy amongst surgeons, pediatricians and anesthesiologists is desirable to facilitate rapid diagnosis and adequate treatment in order to prevent life-threatening situations.

Keywords: tonsillectomy; subcutaneous emphysema; mediastinal emphysema; mediastinitis; complication; bacteremia

1. Introduction

Adenotonsillectomy is one of the most frequently performed surgical procedures in the daily practice of an otorhinolaryngologist, especially in children. Nevertheless, the operation is associated with several severe pre- and post-operative complications. According to literature, primary or secondary bleeding, pain and temporary taste disorders are the most common complications [1–5]. In the Netherlands, according to the national guideline, potential postoperative bleeding and taste disorders are obliged to be mentioned by the otorhinolaryngologist during the pre-operative intake [2,3,6,7]. Other less frequent complications include damage to teeth, otalgia, lingual edema, injury to the glossopharyngeal nerve and injury to the carotid artery [4]. Infectious complications are not frequently reported but can be serious in case of bacteremia [8]. Furthermore, a known but rare and potentially life-threatening complication is the development of (cervico)facial subcutaneous and/or mediastinal emphysema [9–13].

In this case report, we describe the case of a young boy with cervicofacial subcutaneous and mediastinal emphysema after adenotonsillectomy followed by a serious systemic infection caused by group A beta-hemolytic streptococci. We will summarize the current literature on cervicofacial subcutaneous and/or mediastinal emphysema and infectious complications after adenotonsillectomy.

2. Case Report

A 22-month-old boy with Down syndrome was admitted to our department for elective adenotonsillectomy because of sleep apnea due to adenoidal and tonsillar hypertrophy.

Despite conservative treatment for the previous five months with nasal rinsing and intranasal steroid spray, his symptoms had deteriorated and he was indicated for surgery with post-operative observation overnight. Except for the presence of habitual belching, his medical history revealed no other abnormalities.

After a nontraumatic and uneventful orotracheal intubation, guillotine adenotonsillectomy was performed under general anesthesia. Hemostasis was achieved by dry gauze compress on both sides, no bipolar cautery was necessary. Both tonsils were easily removed without remarkable adhesions and there was no excessive bleeding during or after the procedure. Our patient was monitored in the recovery room and discharged to the ward after 40 min.

The next morning during visitation rounds, the patient's dismissal home was postponed due to inadequate fluid intake. The physical examination and vital signs showed no aberrant findings. In the afternoon the patient was reassessed because of a swelling on the right side of his face. His vital signs were normal and there was no fever or difficulty breathing. Further physical examination showed facial swelling on the right side and crepitus was felt during palpation. There were no signs of cellulitis. Oral examination of the tonsil bed revealed normal wound healing without obvious mucosal tears. Ultrasound confirmed the presence of subcutaneous emphysema.

The progression of the emphysema quickly resulted in signs of an obstructed airway with a saturation of 81% SpO2 and the use of accessory muscles of respiration. The patient was quickly transferred to the pediatric intensive care unit where he was intubated. Shortly after successful intubation, the patient went in cardiac arrest and 2 min of cardiopulmonary resuscitation was performed. Bedside evaluation arrest ruled out pneumothorax, cardiac tamponade, hypoxia or airway obstruction and hypovolemia. Cardiac ultasonography showed a diminished ventricular function.

Blood tests showed white blood cell count of 0.78×10^3e/uL and a C-reactive protein of 142 mg/L. Blood cultures were positive with group A beta-hemolytic streptococci. A computed tomography scan (Appendix Figure A1) revealed mediastinal infectious infiltration besides subcutaneous emphysema. In retrospect, the cause of the cardiopulmonary arrest turned out to be due to sepsis/mediastinitis.

Our patient was treated with broad spectrum antibiotics, inotropes and intravenous immunoglobulin. The further course was uneventful. The subcutaneous emphysema resolved over the following days and the patient could be extubated 6 days after admission to the PICU. Finally, 15 days after surgery he was discharged home. Fortunately, follow-up consultations showed no neurological residual symptoms.

3. Discussion

Subcutaneous emphysema has been described in the literature as a complication following tonsillectomy. The seriousness of emphysema varies and includes bilateral cases, pneumomediastinum, pneumothorax and even pneumoperitoneum.

Massive emphysema can compress the trachea, especially in young children, since their tracheal rings are soft. Due to the connection between the parapharyngeal and retropharyngeal space, emphysema can subsequently spread to the mediastinum, causing a pneumomediastinum and even pneumothorax, with major respiratory consequences [14,15]. The typical clinical finding by physical examination is crepitus on palpation. Other diagnoses such as hematoma, allergic reaction or necrotizing fasciitis have to be excluded.

The latter is especially important to distinguish, since rapid treatment with intravenous antibiotics and surgical debridement can be curative. Local tenderness and erythema with variant vital signs are warning signs of infection [16].

It has been suggested that patients with severe adhesions of the tonsil to the superior constrictor muscle, for example after recurrent tonsillitis or peritonsillar abscess, are more prone to develop postoperative subcutaneous emphysema. Due to the adhesions, the dissection of the tonsils from the tonsillar bed can be difficult, increasing the risk of injury to the tonsillar fossa [12]. Accordingly, assuming that removing pediatric tonsils is easier, we found only three cases of pediatric patients with subcutaneous emphysema since 2000, with ages of 6, 7 and 11 years [15,17,18].

Although the exact pathophysiological mechanism is still unknown, "ascending" and "descending" routes are described [9,17,19].

In the ascending mechanism, a rupture occurs anywhere along the tracheobronchial tree from a pre-existing abnormality such as an alveolar bleb or laryngocele or from an acquired defect from traumatic intubation. Following excessive positive pressure ventilation or because of increased intrathoracic pressure, the pre-existing defect can rupture causing the entry of air into the peritracheal or perialveolar tissue. In the case of an alveolar rupture, air can pass through the perivascular sheaths into the mediastinum. Through the subfascial tissue, air can 'ascend' to the subcutaneous tissues of the neck and facial area [17].

In the descending pathway, subcutaneous air infiltration into the pharyngeal space is caused by deep dissection into the tonsil fossa, causing a breach of the superior constrictor muscle and the underlying fascia. Increased intrathoracic pressure (coughing, vomiting, physical exertion, straining and/or manual positive pressure mask ventilation) allows air to migrate through the defect.

Since the subcutaneous emphysema was initially limited to our patient's face and there was a nontraumatic intubation, we consider the 'descending' pathway to be more likely.

The habitual belching also supports the presence of the descending mechanism.

In order to prevent the occurrence of subcutaneous emphysema, it is important to perform careful surgery. In our patient, we performed a tonsillectomy using the Guillotine technique, according to the Dutch guideline. The aim, as in all techniques, is to remove the tonsils completely with minimal hemorrhage and minimal postoperative complications [20]. However, to date there is no international consensus on which technique is best to perform a tonsillectomy. In the case reports describing the development of subcutaneous emphysema, different techniques were used (i.e., electro-dissection with bipolar scissors, tonsil dissector, Ultracision Harmonic scalpel and cold steel elevators). Conclusions about the used technique and its role in the development of subcutaneous emphysema cannot be made. A tonsillotomy (intracapsular, partial or subtotal tonsillectomy), in which the tonsil parenchyma is removed without damage to the tonsillar fossa and the superior constrictor muscle, might minimalize the risk of postoperative subcutaneous emphysema [20,21]. Furthermore, if possible, patients can be instructed to avoid activities that increase intrathoracic pressure. Unfortunately, our patient could not repress the belching.

The treatment of subcutaneous emphysema is mostly conservative but includes broad-spectrum antibiotics to prevent infection from the oral cavity. In case of an evident mucosal rupture, reparation of the damage is recommended. Medication to suppress increasing intrathoracic pressure, such as anti-emetics, codeine or stool softeners can be prescribed [9]. In most cases the subcutaneous emphysema resolves spontaneously and no further treatment is necessary. Of the 43 cases described in a review by Saravakos, three patients needed re-intubation, one patient required temporary tracheostomy to secure their airway and three patients underwent thoracotomy for air drainage out of the mediastinum [9,10,18,22–25].

Our patient was intubated because of progressive, airway-obstructing emphysema, but despite effective airway management he deteriorated due to a systemic infectious disease.

Bacteremia after tonsillectomy has also been described and is relatively innocent in most cases. According to the literature, transient bacteremia occurs in 22% to 70% of all post-tonsillectomy patients and generally ceases within 20 to 40 min in healthy patients [26]. The most commonly responsible micro-organism is the Haemophilus influenza. Although group A beta-hemolytic streptococci are frequently found in local tonsillar oropharyngeal cultures, they are rare in blood cultures and we found only two previous cases describing the presence of a severe systemic group A streptococcal infection in otherwise healthy patients after tonsillectomy. In the first case, a four-year-old girl developed a severe streptococcal septic shock syndrome the night after surgery. In the second case, a four-year-old boy revealed invasive streptococcal infection symptoms 5 days after surgery. He died 4 days after re-admission due to a ruptured mycotic aneurysm of the ascending aorta and hemorrhagic pericarditis caused by group A streptococcal sepsis [8].

Invasive infections with group-A-streptococci can be devastating due to endotoxin release resulting in a septic shock syndrome. The overall mortality of such streptococcal septic shock syndrome is around 50% [27].

Although rare, serious infectious complications after tonsillectomy can occur and should be kept in mind. Prompt recognition and treatment are necessary. Authors should discuss the results and how they can be interpreted in the context of previous studies and of the working hypotheses. The findings and their implications should be discussed in the broadest context possible. Future research directions may also be highlighted.

4. Conclusions

We described a severely complicated clinical course after an uncomplicated adenotonsillectomy. Since the development of subcutaneous emphysema as well as the presence of a group A hemolytic streptococci bacteremia after tonsillectomy are both rare but life-threatening complications, we should all be aware of their (co-)existence. Intensive co-operation by surgeons, pediatricians and anesthesiologists is necessary for fast and adequate diagnosis and treatment to prevent further damage.

Consent for Publication: The patient's parents provided their written informed consent for the publication of the case report.

Author Contributions: Writing—original draft preparation, A.D.; review and editing, G.v.H.; review, editing and supervision, L.V.

Funding: This research received no external funding.

Conflicts of Interest: The authors declare no conflict of interest.

Appendix A

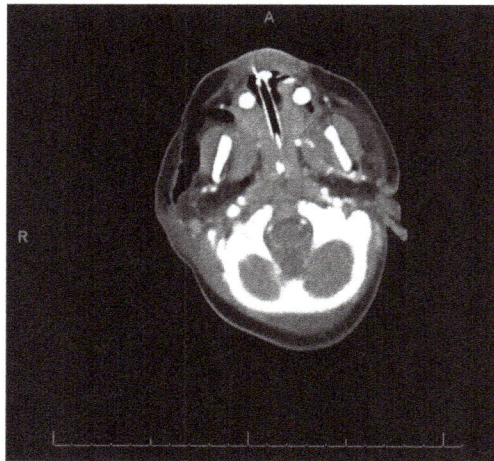

Figure A1. Computed tomography scan of our patient taken two days after the adenotonsillectomy. The image shows infiltrative soft-tissue and subfascial emphysema in the facial region particularly on the right side.

References

1. Greig, S. Current perspectives on the role of tonsillectomy. *J. Paediatr. Child Health* **2017**, *53*, 1065–1070. [CrossRef] [PubMed]

2. Heiser, C.; Basile, N.; Giger, R.; Cao Van, H.; Guinand, N.; Hörmann, K.; Stuck, B.A. Taste Disturbance Following Tonsillectomy—A Prospective Study. *Laryngoscope* **2010**, *120*, 2119–2124. [CrossRef] [PubMed]

3. Heiser, C.; Basile, N.; Giger, R.; Cao Van, H.; Guinand, N.; Hörmann, K.; Stuck, B.A. Taste Disorders after Tonsillectomy: A long-term follow-up. *Laryngoscope* **2012**, *122*, 1265–1266. [CrossRef] [PubMed]

4. De Luca Canto, G.; Pacheco-Pereira, C.; Aydinoz, S.; Bhattacharjee, R.; Tan, H.; Kheirandish-Gozal, L.; Flores-Mir, C.; Gozal, D. Adenotonsillectomy Complications: A Meta-analysis. *Pediatrics* **2015**, *136*, 702–718. [CrossRef] [PubMed]

5. Kendrick, D.; Gibbin, K. An audit of the complications of paediatric tonsillectomy, adenoidectomy and adenotonsillectomy. *Clin. Otolaryngol. Allied Sci.* **1993**, *18*, 115–117. [CrossRef] [PubMed]

6. *Richtlijn Ziekten van Adenoïd en Tonsillen in de Tweede lijn 2014*; Nederlandse Vereniging voor KNO-heelkunde en Heelkunde van het Hoofd-Halsgebied: Utrecht, The Netherlands, 2014.

7. Mistry, D.; Kelly, G. Consent for tonsillectomy. *Clin. Otolaryngol. Allied Sci.* **2004**, *29*, 362–368. [CrossRef] [PubMed]

8. Timmers-Raaijmaakers, B.C.M.S.; Wolfs, T.F.W.; Jansen, N.J.G.; Bos, A.P.; van Vught, A.J. Invasive group A streptococcal infection after tonsillectomy. *Pediatr. Infect. Dis. J.* **2003**, *22*, 929–930. [CrossRef]

9. Saravakos, P.; Taxeidis, M.; Kastanioudakis, I.; Reichel, O. Subcutaneous emphysema as a complication of tonsillectomy: Systematic literature review and case report. *Iran. J. Otorhinolaryngol.* **2018**, *30*, 3–10.

10. Gillot, C.; Tombu, S.; Crestani, V.; Huvelle, P.; Moreau, P. Subcutaneous emphysema and mediastinitis: Unusual complications of tonsillectomy. *B-ENT* **2005**, *1*, 197–200.

11. Panerari, A.C.; Soter, A.C.; Silva, F.L.; Oliveira, L.F.; Neves, M.D.; Cedin, A.C. Onset of subcutaneous emphysema and pneumomediastinum after tonsillectomy: A case report. *Braz. J. Otorhinolaryngol.* **2005**, *71*, 94–96. [CrossRef]

12. Kim, J.P.; Park, J.J.; Kang, H.S.; Song, M.S. Subcutaneous emphysema and pneumomediastinum after tonsillectomy. *Am. J. Otolaryngol.* **2010**, *31*, 212–215. [CrossRef] [PubMed]

13. Tran, D.D.; Littlefield, P.D. Late presentation of subcutaneous emphysema and pneumomediastinum following elective tonsillectomy. *Am. J. Otolaryngol.* **2015**, *36*, 299–302. [CrossRef] [PubMed]

14. Yelnoorkar, S.; Issing, W. Cervicofacial Surgical Emphysema following Tonsillectomy. *Case Rep. Otolaryngol.* **2014**, *2014*, 746152. [CrossRef] [PubMed]

15. Miman, M.C.; Ozturan, O.; Durmus, M.; Kalcioglu, M.; Gedik, E. Cervical subcutaneous emphysema: An usual complication of adenotonsillectomy. *Paediatr. Anaesth.* **2001**, *11*, 491–493. [CrossRef] [PubMed]

16. Sonne, J.E.; Kim, S.B.; Frank, D.K. Cervical necrotizing fasciitis as a complication of tonsillectomy. *Otolaryngol. Head Neck Surg.* **2001**, *125*, 670–672. [CrossRef] [PubMed]

17. Shine, N.P.; Sader, C.; Coates, H. Cervicofacial emphysema and pneumomediastinum following pediatric adenotonsillectomy: A rare complication. *Int. J. Pediatr. Otorhinolaryngol.* **2005**, *69*, 1579–1582. [CrossRef] [PubMed]

18. Piotrowski, S.; Jesikiewicz, D. Mediastinal emphysema as a complication of the tonsilloadenotomy in child. *Otolaryngol. Pol.* **2009**, *63*, 528–531. [CrossRef]

19. Ero, O.; Aydin, E. A Rare Complication of Tonsillectomy: Subcutaneous Emphysema. *Turk. Arch. Otorhinolaryngol.* **2016**, *54*, 172–174.

20. Frampton, S.J.; Ward, M.J.A.; Sunkaraneni, V.S.; Ismail-Koch, H.; Sheppard, Z.A.; Salib, R.J.; Jain, P.K. Guillotine versus dissection tonsillectomy: Randomized controlled trial. *J. Laryngol. Otol.* **2012**, *126*, 1142–1149. [CrossRef]

21. Smith, S. Tonsillotomy: An alternative surgical option to total tonsillectomy in children with obstructive sleep apnoea. *Aus. Fam. Physician* **2016**, *45*, 894–896.

22. Hung, M.H.; Shih, P.Y.; Yang, Y.M.; Lan, J.Y.; Fan, S.Z.; Jeng, C.S. Cervicofacial subcutaneous emphysema following tonsillectomy: Implications for anesthesiologists. *Acta Anaesthesiol. Taiwan* **2009**, *47*, 134–137. [CrossRef]

23. Stewart, A.E.; Brewster, D.F.; Bernstein, P.E. Subcutaneous emphysema and pneumomediastinum complication tonsillectomy. *Arch. Otolaryngol. Head Neck Surg.* **2004**, *130*, 1324–1327. [CrossRef] [PubMed]

24. Ferguson, C.C.; McGarry, G.P.; Beckman, I.H.; Brder, M. Surgical emphysema complicating tonsillectomy and dental extraction. *Can. Med. Assoc. J.* **1955**, *72*, 847–848. [PubMed]

25. Pratt, L.W.; Hornberger, H.R.; Moore, V.J. Mediastinal emphysema complicating tonsillectomy and adenoidectomy. *Ann. Otol. Rhinol. Laryngol.* **1962**, *71*, 158–169. [CrossRef] [PubMed]

26. Klug, T.E.; Henriksen, J.; Rusan, M.; Fuursted, K.; Ovesen, T. Bacteremia during quinsy and elective tonsillectomy: An evaluation of antibiotic prophylaxis recommendations for patients undergoing tonsillectomy. *J. Cardiovasc. Pharmacol. Ther.* **2012**, *17*, 298–302. [CrossRef] [PubMed]

27. Low, D.E. Toxic shock syndrome: Major advances in pathogenesis, but not treatment. *Crit. Care Clin.* **2013**, *29*, 651–675. [CrossRef]

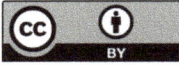

Review

Fine Needle Aspiration Cytology for Neck Masses in Childhood. An Illustrative Approach

Consolato Sergi *, Aneesh Dhiman and Jo-Ann Gray

Department of Lab. Medicine and Pathology, University of Alberta, 8440 112 St., Edmonton,
AB T6G 2B7, Canada; Aneesh.Dhiman@albertahealthservices.ca (A.D.); grayj@telus.net (J.-A.G.)
* Correspondence: sergi@ualberta.ca

Received: 29 January 2018; Accepted: 19 April 2018; Published: 22 April 2018

Abstract: The primary indication of fine-needle aspiration cytology of the head and neck region is a thyroid nodule or a mass located in the cervical area or the head. Although a thyroid nodule may raise the suspicion of malignancy, less than one in 20 cases results in a carcinoma. In addition, the list of differential diagnoses is quite different according to the age of the patient. A number of benign lesions, such as branchial cysts, sialadenosis, and sialoadenitis are often seen in childhood and youth. The malignant lesions that are on the top of the list of a pediatric mass of the head and neck (H&N) region include rhabdomyosarcoma, neuroblastoma, and papillary carcinoma of the thyroid gland. This critical review of the diagnostic features of a pediatric mass of the H&N region is accompanied by panels of several cytology features that may be of help to the cytopathologist and clinician.

Keywords: cytopathology; head and neck; children

1. Introduction

In the era of transcriptomics and advancements identified at increasing pace in this 2nd decade of the 3rd millennium, an apparently simple approach with a needle, a slide, and some staining tools may be awkward. It seems that the fine needle aspiration biopsy was performed first in 1857, although several techniques and new protocols have transformed this seemingly simple procedure into a practice that is impressively diffuse worldwide. Aside from scarring in some patients, there are complications due to unnecessary surgery which is well known to many pediatricians. In adults, fine needle aspiration cytology (FNAC) has been used with great success as the primary screening test for thyroid nodules [1–3]. In non-thyroid nodules, FNAC has also increased rates of sensitivity and specificity in numerous studies [4]. However, such a structured approach has remained unused in the evaluation of pediatric nodules and instead, urgent analysis using scalpel and surgery is performed. This critical review of the literature highlights the information we can receive using FNAC in pediatrics and shows some illustrative cytologic features that may be extremely useful for both training or experienced cytologists and pediatricians. The present study was designed to critically review the role of FNAC and its utility in pediatric head and neck (H&N) lesions. It is not a comprehensive atlas and has no aim to fill all gaps of the H&N lesions in pediatrics, which are covered in excellent texts and books. Nevertheless, our paper emphasizes the procedure and specifies the spectrum of the H&N lesions in the pediatric age group, highlighting some studies gathered from the literature comparing cytology and histology of the H&N lesions.

2. Methodology

A neck mass that is resistant to antibiotics for more than four weeks should be considered the primary indication to proceed with non-thyroid FNAC. Other signs should also include cases of asymmetric benign lymphadenopathy as well as cervical lymph nodal enlargement showing unusual location, fast expansion, evidence of weight loss or loss of appetite, and night sweats. The identification of skin changes and/or a fixed/immobile mass may favor a malignant lesion and is also an indication to proceed with FNAC. An FNAC with a critical result may often be managed in our institution within a few hours planning for surgery to be performed in the same day or the day after. Nonthyroidal FNAC should be conducted while keeping in mind that the patient may be a potential surgical candidate. Other indications for an FNAC may involve an atypical presentation with systemic symptoms; the urgency made clear by the medical team or family and the willingness to diagnose the lesion before the typical 2–7 days of surgical processing. In consideration of the high percentage of papillary thyroid carcinomas in childhood and youth, FNAC should be offered as the first procedure for all pediatric thyroid nodules following an ultrasound scan showing a lesion with a diameter of 1 cm or more. In the case of pediatric thyroid nodules with lesions measuring less than 1 cm in diameter, an FNAC with a critical result processing (same day or day after or within 24 h) should be offered in the event that concerning ultrasonographic results are present. Ultrasound anomalies will include hypoechogenicity, irregularity of the margins, or increased vascularity of the lesion. FNAC is usually performed in the Otolaryngology/ear-nose-throat (ENT) clinical department or inpatient ward by specialized and well-trained personnel, including a cytopathologist, an interventional radiologist, or a (pediatric) surgeon. Topical (4% lidocaine cream) anesthesia is used with some general low sedation, and all biopsies should be performed using image guidance. In our opinion, the practice to use palpation should be discouraged or left to very palpable nodules to reduce the annual false negativity rate [5–7]. The procedure involves the use of a 25- to 27-gauge needle, and a range of 3 to 5 passes are performed for each targeted site, representing a single FNA procedure. If a patient has multiple targeted nodules or masses, various aspirates are usually performed at the discretion of the medical personnel. The aspiration of the material is then used for smear preparation, which includes air-dried slides stained with Diff-Quik and alcohol-fixed slides stained with the Papanicolaou stain. It is paramount to perform additional testing at the same time to avoid unnecessary delay in the diagnosis. In fact, residual material is typically used for ThinPrep processing (Hologic Inc., Marlborough, MA, USA), microbiology, and molecular biology studies. To confirm whether the material is adequate in a lymph node, a small drop of the aspirate is placed onto the preparation slides for immediate assessment (also technically labelled 'rapid on-site evaluation'), while the remainder is rinsed in a cell preservative. Typically, 10 million cells are considered adequate for cytopathology assessment, which requires 2–3 passes indeed.

The cell block preparation is routinely performed in our institution and not only in case of ambiguous interpretation of the aspirates. It is also important to advise the lab technician to stain some tissue sections of the cell block with hematoxylin-eosin and keep some unstained tissue sections for histochemical (special) stains, immunohistochemical stains, and further ancillary testing as required. The cytology aspirates are interpreted initially by a cytotechnologist and subsequently by a pediatric pathologist with an intra-institutional cytopathology consultation adjured by a cytopathologist. FNAC cases receive diagnoses with an adequacy interpretation (unsatisfactory, satisfactory), a primary interpretation (nondiagnostic, negative for malignant cells, atypical cells present, suspicious for cancerous cells, or positive for malignant cells), and a free text explanatory diagnosis. The category 'less than optimal' is not often used in our institutions to avoid non-categorical decisions.

It is also advisable to perform a yearly outcome rating using spreadsheet-based correlation to surgical histopathology and clinical follow-up. In the case of clinical monitoring, laboratory values and clinical presentation are part of a 6-month–1-year follow-up, while surgical histopathology, which is based on either an incisional surgical biopsy or an excisional surgical biopsy, is considered the reference standard in the diagnosis of tumors of the H&N region. In the setting of a quality assurance program, true positives are cytopathologic results that warrant surgical treatment and are confirmed as such using surgical histopathologic biopsy. True negatives are cytopathologic results that did not designate a need for surgery and are established as such using the surgical histopathologic biopsy. Clinical true negatives are negative conditions on cytology that resolve or did not progress without surgical intervention. In case of false positives cytology, cytopathology results are positive, but there would have been no need for surgical treatment, while false negatives are unremarkable cytopathologic results without a need for surgery, although a surgical intervention would have been the right option. To avoid bias in any cytology-pathology correlation quality assurance program, it is prudent that pathologists interpreting surgical histopathology slides are distinct from cytopathologists interpreting the FNAC. Some infective or non-malignant conditions, such as atypical mycobacterial infection, cervicofacial abscess, or lymphatic malformations, may require surgical diagnosis or treatment but may also appropriately be managed by medical therapy. If the appropriate medical treatment is initiated and results efficacious and efficient, the result is labeled as an actual clinical positive. The 2015 Standards for Reporting of Diagnostic Accuracy (STARD) guideline for reporting diagnostic accuracy studies should be used [8].

In the setting of procedure complications, care should be taken when considering the side effects of FNAC, e.g., infection and damage to nearby structures. By reviewing the literature, we found a limited core of evidence for such side effects if a safe procedure is applied. In particular, an honest and straightforward report provided by Chen et al. [9], who reported a 19-year-old girl with a painful goiter, which became more painful after fine needle aspiration (FNA). The patient's second FNAC revealed only many neutrophils and an antibiotic treatment improved the pain, but the goiter persisted. The third FNA revealed cytology of papillary carcinoma cells and the total thyroidectomy showed ischemic necrosis with neutrophilic aggregation around the needle track other than a papillary thyroid carcinoma. This report reveals the possibility of missing malignant cells in a background of an infection following an improper FNA. Secondary infection and ischemic necrosis may indeed occur after FNA, and aseptic procedures are necessary to prevent bacteria from seeding into the thyroid gland. Disinfection of the FNAC site and experienced personnel are mandatory for laboratories that harbor periodic accreditation by the College of the American Pathologists (CAP) operating in healthcare institutions in United States of America and Canada. Thus, side effects may occur following an FNA procedure. Nevertheless, we consider that FNAC in children and adolescents is accurate, safe, and well-accepted in a wide range of lesions of the head and neck regions. A CAP accreditation or a similar accreditation outside of North America should be requested by all pediatricians and parents of the affected child.

3. Diagnostics

In most of the cases, FNAC of the H&N region is performed to investigate clinically suspicious lymphadenopathy, and the primary differential diagnoses include congenital anomaly, reactive/infectious lymphadenopathy, lymphoma, and metastatic disease, but also thyroid gland disease and salivary gland disease.

3.1. Congenital Lesion

The age is also particularly important to keep in mind, and 75% of branchial cysts occur in 20–40 year-old patients [10–14]. Benign squamous-lined cysts are usually characterized by abundant inflammatory cells (neutrophils), with few unremarkable squamous epithelial cells with bland nuclear features, and cholesterol crystals, while a large number of squamous cells with or without occasional nuclear hyperchromasia, nuclear membrane irregularity, and high nucleus to cytoplasm ratio portend for a malignant diagnosis.

3.2. Reactive/Infectious Lymphadenopathy and Malignant Lymphoma

In about 2/3 of cases, de novo lymphadenopathies of the H&N region are benign, and even a history of malignancy present in a child with a de novo lymphadenopathy will have a rate of benignancy probably approaching half of the cases [15,16]. Moreover, additional surgical procedures have been avoided in up to 61% of cases in one review [17]. The cytopathological diagnosis of reactive is mostly accurate in children and youth with less in 1 out of 20 (~5%) subsequent (false-negative) malignant diagnoses [2,18]. Cytologic features of reactive lymphadenopathy include polymorphic lymphoid cells showing a clear-cut sequence of maturation, prominent reactive cells arising from germinal centers, the presence of tingible body macrophages, the lack of a monomorphic lymphoid population and the simultaneous presence of a variegated (non-homogeneous) cell population smear, and the lack of a subpopulation (even minimal) of large, irregular lymphoid cells potentially indicative of Hodgkin's lymphoma, anaplastic T-cell lymphoma, large B-cell lymphoma). Necrotizing granulomata are often characteristic of underlying tuberculous infection (particularly systemic), although they may also be found in fungal infection and other acid-fast bacilli (AFB) (e.g., mycobacteria causing scrofula). In a child, the finding of granulomata may suggest non-tuberculous AFB, especially in a child, and cat-scratch disease should be considered in this age group. Granulomas without evidence of necrosis are suggestive of sarcoidosis, toxoplasmosis, or foreign-body giant cell reaction. In all cases, a thorough microbiological investigation is paramount (e.g., *Bartonella henselae* for cat-scratch disease). The correlation between clinical and laboratory findings using electronic medical charts or liaising with the clinician is essential. In fact, serological tests may be useful in a subset of cases for differentiating systemic lupus erythematosus lymphadenitis from Kikuchi–Fujimoto's disease, which is histiocytic necrotizing lymphadenitis. Finally, it is important not to forget that a florid granulomatous pattern can mislead the cytopathologist disguising both Hodgkin's lymphoma and Non-Hodgkin's lymphoma.

3.3. Rhabdomyosarcoma and Neuroblastoma

In a pediatric setting, the most fearful malignant diagnoses in the H&N region, apart from malignant lymphoma, are rhabdomyosarcoma and neuroblastoma. Rhabdomyosarcoma is considered to harbor three main subtypes, including embryonal, which is the most frequent type, the alveolar, and the pleomorphic, which most commonly seen in adults. Rhabdomyosarcoma occurs very often in the head and neck region and the extremities, with the trunk reserved for the third location. Cytomorphology features of the embryonal rhabdomyosarcoma include a variability of patterns including round to spindle-shaped cells, some pleomorphism (different from the marked pleomorphism of the pleomorphic type of the rhabdomyosarcoma of the adult), a variable number of rhabdomyoblasts may be the distinctive clue for the cytopathologist, and, occasionally, inclusion-like cytoplasmic condensation, which is also known as myogenic differentiation [18]. Rhabdomyoblastic differentiation is characterized by elongated, strap- or tadpole-shaped cytoplasm, and nuclear eccentricity. The nuclear diagnostic clues also rely on dense hyperchromatic chromatin and nuclear membrane irregularity (Figure 1a,b). The alveolar rhabdomyosarcoma is distinctively identified by larger, uniformly round to variably polygonal cells with an increased number of mitotic figures in the background with scattered rhabdomyoblasts and giant cells with wreath-like nuclei. Metastatic neuroblastoma to the neck is quite rare in adulthood, but it is a principal differential diagnosis in infants and children, especially in infants. Although most neuroblastomas arise in the adrenal gland or the paravertebral sympathetic chain bilaterally, this pediatric tumor can occur anywhere along the sympathetic chain. Cytomorphology of neuroblastoma may be entirely different according to the degree of ganglionic differentiation of the neuroblastoma. These features include a fibrillary matrix, dyshesive small undifferentiated cells, sparse Homer–Wright rosettes, a nuclear pattern labeled as "salt and pepper" for the variability of the granularity of the nuclear chromatin, and, occasionally, ganglion-like cells (Figure 1c,d). In rare occasions, necrotic debris and dysmorphic calcifications are seen [18]. It is paramount to distinguish reactive/reparative changes from the diagnoses mentioned above [19] (Figure 1e,f). A spectrum of appearance needs to be kept in mind in case of benign fibrous proliferation. The retention of a low nucleus to cytoplasm ratio is crucial in case of prior radiation where cells may be large, showing irregularity of the nuclei, multinucleation, all features that may be quite worrisome. In fact, the resolution may decrease the inflammatory background, making the diagnosis particularly distressful for an inexperienced pathologist. Moreover, the myofibroblasts that occur in benign fibrous proliferations may become slender with less conspicuous nucleoli during the healing process. In all cases, the identification of pleomorphism, nuclear hyperchromasia, high nucleus to cytoplasm ratio, and atypical mitoses suggest malignancy that needs to be surgically acted upon as soon as possible.

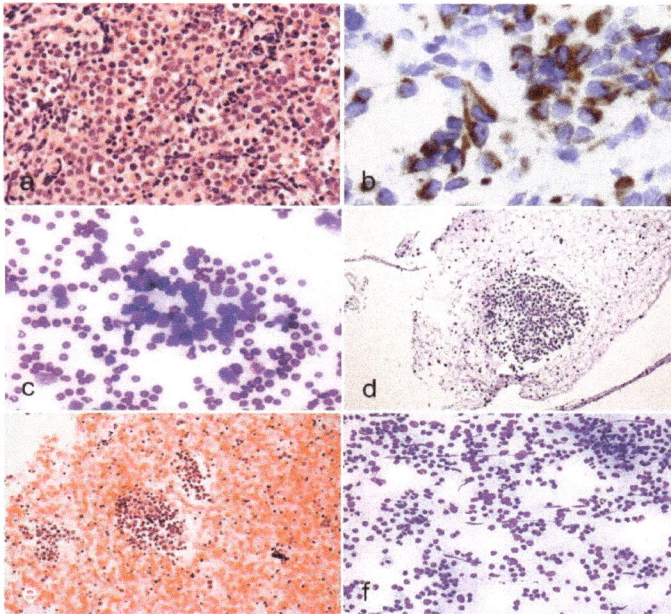

Figure 1. (**a,b**) Rhabdomyosarcoma cytology in cell block (Papanicolaou, ×200) and smears fixed and immunostained with the antibody anti-desmin (Avidin-Biotin-Complex immunostaining, ×630). (**c,d**) Neuroblastoma cytology in smears and cell block showing hyperchromatic cells with high nucleus to cytoplasm ratio (Diff-Quik, ×100 and ×100, **c** and **d**, respectively). (**e,f**) Reactive changes of soft tissue showing a mixture of cells with variable morphology (cell block and smears stained with Papanicolaou and Diff-Quik, ×100 and ×100, **e** and **f**, respectively).

3.4. Thyroid Gland Disease

The introduction of synoptic reports has been crucial in improving healthcare worldwide, allowing a common platform for adequately assessing patients with neoplastic disease. Thyroid cases receive an adequacy interpretation, a first interpretation using "The Bethesda System for Reporting Thyroid Cytopathology" (TBSRTC), and a free text explanatory diagnosis with a comment according to the pathologist or cytopathologist [2]. It is also encouraged that the cytopathologist or the pathologist liaise with the clinical team in case an FNAC may indicate suspicious malignant cells or some distinct cancerous cells. TBSRTC categories include insufficient for diagnosis, benign, atypical cells of undetermined significance, suspicious for a follicular neoplasm, suspicious for a Hürthle cell neoplasm, suspicious for malignancy (papillary carcinoma, medullary carcinoma, lymphoma, metastatic tumor, other), and malignant. Despite iodine supplementation, multinodular goiter (MNG) occurs in North America. MNG is a common disorder of the thyroid gland with multiple nodules [18]. The macrofollicular pattern of a follicular neoplasm is indistinguishable from MNG Cytologically, a benign follicular nodule shows mainly macrofollicles, low/moderate cellularity, cohesive follicular cells with uniformity and even spacing, coarse chromatin, as well as colloid, which may be copious. The differential diagnosis of benign follicular nodules includes suspicious follicular nodule, suspicious Hürthle cell nodule, and papillary carcinoma. In some benign nodules, focal cytologic atypia may be present and becomes a diagnostic challenge. Of note, Hürthle cell metaplasia is often seen in MNG and the cells may show at places marked nuclear atypia. Hashimoto or chronic lymphocytic thyroiditis is characterized by a mixed population of lymphocytes, tingible-body macrophages, dendritic-lymphocytic clusters, Hürthle cells and scant colloid. Hyperplastic Hürthle cells nodules may occur in Hashimoto thyroiditis mimicking a Hürthle cell tumor [18]. The differential diagnosis of Hashimoto thyroiditis includes a reactive lymph node, MNG with predominant Hürthle cell change, primary malignant lymphoma of the thyroid gland, Hürthle cell neoplasm, and papillary thyroid carcinoma. A subacute thyroiditis and Riedel disease are not a common event in pediatric age or youth. The category of suspicious for a follicular neoplasm has some cytologic features including marked cellularity, scant colloid, predominant microfollicles or epithelial trabeculae, and enlarged, crowded follicular cells (differently from the uniformity and even spacing of the benign lesions) [18]. In a pediatric setting, a suspicious for a follicular neoplasm poses a differential diagnosis of a benign follicular nodule, papillary thyroid carcinoma, and parathyroid adenoma or carcinoma. Other malignant masses have other distinguishing features in childhood and youth. A suspicious for Hürthle cell neoplasm diagnosis has cytologic features showing an almost complete cell population of Hürthle cells, usually dyshesive cells with prominent nucleolus, and pseudopsammoma bodies. Cytological features of papillary thyroid carcinoma include sheets, microfollicles, and papillae, although the nuclear changes need to be searched carefully. The nuclear changes include grooves, pseudoinclusions, "powdery" chromatin, and thickened and irregular nuclear membrane. There is also nuclear crowding or molding. Cells show a variable amount of cytoplasm and psammoma bodies may be present. The differential diagnosis of papillary carcinoma includes a benign follicular nodule, a follicular neoplasm, Hashimoto thyroiditis, radiotherapy effect, and a hyalinizing trabecular tumor. Although the anaplastic carcinoma does not play any role in childhood or youth, an important entity to keep in mind is the medullary carcinoma. Cytologically, this endocrine parafollicular cells derived tumor shows numerous isolated cells, loose aggregates of cells with epithelioid, plasmacytoid, or spindle-shaped morphology, nuclear changes (rounding or elongation, granularity of the chromatin, inconspicuous nucleolus, pseudoinclusions, and multiple nuclei), cytoplasmic changes (red granules) on Diff-Quik stained preparations, and amyloid. Although rare, two primary malignant lymphomas of the thyroid gland need to be kept in mind and include the diffuse large B cell lymphoma and the extra-nodal marginal zone B-cell lymphoma.

3.5. Salivary Gland Disease

Salivary gland lesions are rare in children, although an increase of salivary gland disease in adolescence and youth has been reported recently [20–22]. Previous research has shown that salivary gland tumors are rare in the young population, but the incidence of all primary salivary gland carcinomas increased with increasing patient age, particularly in patients younger than 30 years. Lesions of the major cephalic salivary glands, with the exception of mumps and cytomegaly, are unusual in children and adolescents, but these lesions may give rise to some different tentative diagnoses [23–25]. Since malignant salivary gland tumors are relatively more frequently recognized in younger patients, a safe approach is advisable, and intradepartmental consultation is crucial. Cytologic diagnoses of malignant tumors are confirmed histologically in 93% of cases, while benign tumor diagnoses are confirmed on histology in 95% of cases. Inflammatory lesions are confirmed on histology in 73%, while benign salivary gland tissue is ascertained as such histologically in 18% of cases [26]. Non-rare malignant salivary gland tumors in childhood and youth are a mucoepidermoid carcinoma, adenoid cystic carcinoma, acinic cell carcinoma, malignant lymphomas, and metastatic tumors from a tumor of the H&N region or paraganglia (e.g., neuroblastoma). Benign neoplasms include pleomorphic adenoma and Warthin's tumor (Figure 2a,b). In childhood, 80–90% of all malignant salivary gland tumors are constituted by mucoepidermoid carcinomas, adenoid-cystic carcinomas, and acinic cell carcinomas.

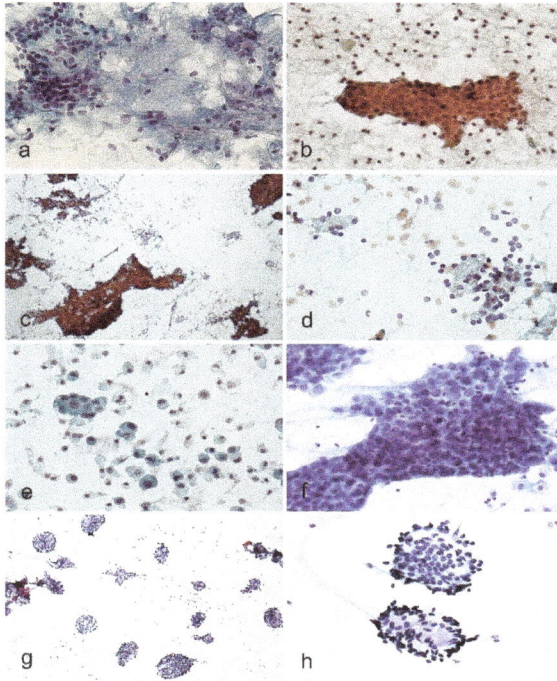

Figure 2. (**a**,**b**) Pleomorphic adenoma and Warthin tumor (Papanicolaou stain, ×100 and ×100, **a** and **b**, respectively). (**c**,**d**) Acinic cell carcinoma (Papanicolaou stain, ×40 and ×100, **c** and **d**, respectively). (**e**,**f**) Mucoepidermoid carcinoma (Papanicolaou stain, ×400 and Papanicolaou stain, ×400, **e** and **f**, respectively). The mucin in the background and the nuclear detail are supportive of a diagnosis of mucoepidermoid carcinoma. (**g**,**h**) Adenoid cystic carcinoma (Diff-Quik, ×100 and ×100, **g** and **h**, respectively). For the details of the single salivary gland tumors, please refer to the text.

In adults, the corresponding figure is only 45% [23]. Despite the low incidence of 15–25% of malignant neoplasms for adults identified in 1969 [27], in a study carried out on 2632 patients following teams and investigations reported a significantly higher relative proportion in young patients [23]. Acinic cell carcinoma is characterized by a hypercellular aspirate with a clean background with tumor cells seen in disorganized clusters with loss of round groupings and lack of an associated ductal epithelium and on higher magnification cells show some uniformity resembling normal serous acinar cells with the cytoplasm being foamy or bubbly and harboring fine dark granules (Figure 2c,d) [28,29]. The examination of the background highlights many naked nuclei. Apart from clear cell tumors, mainly low-grade mucoepidermoid carcinoma and epithelial-myoepithelial carcinoma), oncocytic tumors, sialadenosis, and normal salivary gland tissue need to be kept in the differential diagnosis list. Smears of mucoepidermoid carcinoma are usually low in cellularity with a particularly striking dirty background of mucin and debris. In the smears, the presence of scattered cell clusters of intermediate cells with overlapping epithelial groups, some mucin-coated cells (goblet-cells-like), and few squamous epithelial cells are particularly evident features for the diagnosis of mucoepidermoid carcinoma (Figure 2e,f). However, both components may be quite bland or missing in one or all slides. According to the grade of differentiation, nuclear features may vary from bland to hyperchromasia with a high nucleus to cytoplasm ratio, although this tumor is usually low-grade in childhood and adolescence. Some potential pitfalls in diagnosing the mucoepidermoid carcinoma are some cystic nature of these tumors, which may harvest only hypocellular (even acellular in some cases) mucoid material [30]. Moreover, extracellular mucin is typically copious, mimicking the fibrillary stroma seen in pleomorphic adenomas, although the mucin of pleomorphic adenomas stains less intensely and has no fibrillary pattern. Finally, squamous metaplasia is not only characteristic of mucoepidermoid carcinoma but may be found in other tumors, such as pleomorphic adenoma and Warthin's tumor (Figure 2a,b). The adenoid cystic carcinoma features are large globules of extracellular matrix with or without surrounding basaloid cells. In FNAs with a predominance of basaloid tumor cells, both benign and malignant salivary gland tumors of epithelial–myoepithelial differentiation should be considered in the differential diagnosis (Figure 2g,h) [28,29]. If TBSRTC has received a warming acceptance in many countries, the Milan System for Reporting Salivary Gland Cytology (MSRSGC) seems that will have similar success in the coming years [31–35]. The MSRSGC is an evidence-based tiered classification system that comprises six diagnostic categories associated with an average risk of malignancy (ROM) and clinical management strategies (Table 1). It is expected that the MSRSGC will improve communication between the cytopathologist and the treating pediatrician, facilitating cytologic-histologic correlation, and lead to overall improved patient care.

Table 1. Milan System for Reporting Salivary Gland Cytology (adapted from [36]).

Category significance
Category I => Nondiagnostic, harboring a ROM of 25%
Category II => Nonneoplastic, harboring a ROM of 10%
Category III => Atypia of undetermined significance, harboring an estimated ROM of 20%
Category IV => Neoplasm
Subcategory IVA => Benign, harboring a ROM of <5%
Subcategory IVB => Salivary gland neoplasm of uncertain malignant potential, harboring a ROM of 35%
Category V => Suspicious for malignancy, harboring a ROM of 60%
Category VI => Malignant, harboring a ROM of 90%

Notes: ROM, risk of malignancy.

4. Study Comparison

FNAC is now being considered as a valuable diagnostic aid in many children's hospitals across continents, not only in North America. In most studies, FNAC reveals good aspects, showing the early availability of results, its simplicity, minimal trauma or injury, and the low rate of complications. Ancillary techniques, including flow cytometry, cytogenetics, immunohistochemistry on the cell block, and electron microscopy can be easily applied for the characterization of tumors [20,21,37,38]. Furthermore, FNA does not usually need heavy sedation, and general anesthesia is not necessary. FNAC of the H&N region is a well-accepted technique that has high specificity in most studies [21]. In Table 2, a comparison of four studies is provided.

Table 2. Study Comparison (adapted from [21]).

Study	Rapkiewicz [37]	Jain [20]	Handa [38]	Mittra [21]
Topics	H&N lesions	H&N lesions	Cervical LNs	H&N lesions
Cases	85	748	692 (584 LNs)	100
Age group	0–18 years	0–12 years	0–14 years	0–15 years
Adequacy	N.A.	94%	93.4%	93%
Common site	LN (69.4%)	LN (81%)	LN (84.3%)	LN (87%)
Benign	83%	98.5%	98.5%	88.2%
Malignant	17%	1.5%	1.5%	11.8%

Notes: H&N, Head and Neck; LN, lymph nodes; N.A., not available.

5. Limitations

Most of the studies have several limitations that are inherent in their retrospective nature. First, the lack of standardization of the enrolled patients is reflective of both the diversity of pediatric nodules and the variable diagnostic and treatment approaches of different clinical and surgical teams [17]. In fact, there is often a significant variation in the use, duration, and timing of antibiotic treatment, and the accessibility of the clinical and surgical services was also variable and change over time was present in most of the retrospective studies. The lack of universal follow-up is also an essential drawback of numerous FNAC studies. The importance of the monitoring may be enshrined for all patients with negative FNAC results that need to be instructed to follow up if the mass persists, increases in size, or any concerns remain.

6. Conclusions

The potential avoidance of surgery with associated scarring, early and late septic and non-septic surgical complications, general anesthetic risk, recovery time, and significant expense bills have all been heralded as benefits of FNAC, especially given the high prevalence of non-neoplastic pediatric tumor and masses of the H&N region. FNAC shows an impressive diagnostic accuracy in numerous studies. FNAC is supported by an active lab safety profile and carries a very limited number of drawbacks considering that in the case of a dubious cytology result, a surgery can be planned in a very short time identifying FNAC as a useful triage procedure. In conclusion, FNAC is a safe, well-tolerated, and accurate tool for diagnosing pediatric masses of thyroid and non-thyroid origin in childhood and youth. FNAC plays a vital role in giving comfort to obviate the need for unnecessary immediate surgery in benign nodules (congenital/reactive/inflammatory) and plan a primary surgical intervention in malignant lesions. In consideration of significant health care changes worldwide, we would like to strongly emphasize that when such a triage of pediatric masses of the H&N region is handled, there is a potential decrease in both surgical morbidity and health care costs.

Acknowledgments: We are very grateful to the Women and Children's Health Research Institute (WCHRI) for funding pediatric pathology program at the University of Alberta. C. Sergi has received WCHRI funding for pediatric pathology research programs at the Stollery Children's Hospital, Edmonton, Alberta, Canada.

Author Contributions: Consolato Sergi: study design, data acquisition, analysis and interpretation, manuscript drafting, final manuscript approval; Aneesh Dhiman: study design, data acquisition and interpretation, manuscript revision, final manuscript approval; Jo-Ann Gray: data interpretation, manuscript revision, final manuscript approval.

Conflicts of Interest: The authors declare no conflict of interest.

References

1. Pitman, M.B.; Abele, J.; Ali, S.Z.; Duick, D.; Elsheikh, T.M.; Jeffrey, R.B.; Powers, C.N.; Randolph, G.; Renshaw, A.; Scoutt, L. Techniques for thyroid FNA: A synopsis of the national cancer institute thyroid fine-needle aspiration state of the science conference. *Diagn. Cytopathol.* **2008**, *36*, 407–424. [CrossRef] [PubMed]

2. Cibas, E.S.; Alexander, E.K.; Benson, C.B.; De Agustin, P.P.; Doherty, G.M.; Faquin, W.C.; Middleton, W.D.; Miller, T.; Raab, S.S.; White, M.L.; et al. Indications for thyroid FNA and pre-FNA requirements: A synopsis of the national cancer institute thyroid fine-needle aspiration state of the science conference. *Diagn. Cytopathol.* **2008**, *36*, 390–399. [CrossRef] [PubMed]

3. Abati, A. The national cancer institute thyroid FNA state of the science conference: "Wrapped up". *Diagn. Cytopathol.* **2008**, *36*, 388–389. [CrossRef] [PubMed]

4. Goret, C.C.; Goret, N.E.; Ozdemir, Z.T.; Ozkan, E.A.; Dogan, M.; Yanik, S.; Gumrukcu, G.; Aker, F.V. Diagnostic value of fine needle aspiration biopsy in non-thyroidal head and neck lesions: A retrospective study of 866 aspiration materials. *Int. J. Clin. Exp. Pathol.* **2015**, *8*, 8709–8716. [PubMed]

5. Francis, G.L.; Waguespack, S.G.; Bauer, A.J.; Angelos, P.; Benvenga, S.; Cerutti, J.M.; Dinauer, C.A.; Hamilton, J.; Hay, I.D.; Luster, M.; et al. Management guidelines for children with thyroid nodules and differentiated thyroid cancer. *Thyroid* **2015**, *25*, 716–759. [CrossRef] [PubMed]

6. LaFranchi, S.H. Inaugural management guidelines for children with thyroid nodules and differentiated thyroid cancer: Children are not small adults. *Thyroid* **2015**, *25*, 713–715. [CrossRef] [PubMed]
7. Lim-Dunham, J.E.; Erdem Toslak, I.; Alsabban, K.; Aziz, A.; Martin, B.; Okur, G.; Longo, K.C. Ultrasound risk stratification for malignancy using the 2015 American thyroid association management guidelines for children with thyroid nodules and differentiated thyroid cancer. *Pediatr. Radiol.* **2017**, *47*, 429–436. [CrossRef] [PubMed]
8. Bossuyt, P.M.; Reitsma, J.B.; Bruns, D.E.; Gatsonis, C.A.; Glasziou, P.P.; Irwig, L.; Lijmer, J.G.; Moher, D.; Rennie, D.; de Vet, H.C.; et al. STARD 2015: An updated list of essential items for reporting diagnostic accuracy studies. *BMJ* **2015**, *351*, h5527. [CrossRef] [PubMed]
9. Chen, H.W.; Tseng, F.Y.; Su, D.H.; Chang, Y.L.; Chang, T.C. Secondary infection and ischemic necrosis after fine needle aspiration for a painful papillary thyroid carcinoma: A case report. *Acta Cytol.* **2006**, *50*, 217–220. [CrossRef] [PubMed]
10. Layfield, L.J.; Cibas, E.S.; Baloch, Z. Thyroid fine needle aspiration cytology: A review of the national cancer institute state of the science symposium. *Cytopathology* **2010**, *21*, 75–85. [CrossRef] [PubMed]
11. Layfield, L.J.; Cibas, E.S.; Gharib, H.; Mandel, S.J. Thyroid aspiration cytology: Current status. *CA Cancer J. Clin.* **2009**, *59*, 99–110. [CrossRef] [PubMed]
12. Layfield, L.J.; Abrams, J.; Cochand-Priollet, B.; Evans, D.; Gharib, H.; Greenspan, F.; Henry, M.; LiVolsi, V.; Merino, M.; Michael, C.W.; et al. Post-thyroid FNA testing and treatment options: A synopsis of the national cancer institute thyroid fine needle aspiration state of the science conference. *Diagn. Cytopathol.* **2008**, *36*, 442–448. [CrossRef] [PubMed]
13. Layfield, L.J. Fine-needle aspiration in the diagnosis of head and neck lesions: A review and discussion of problems in differential diagnosis. *Diagn. Cytopathol.* **2007**, *35*, 798–805. [CrossRef] [PubMed]
14. Layfield, L.J. Fine-needle aspiration biopsy in the diagnosis of pediatric tumors. *West. J. Med.* **1991**, *154*, 90–91. [PubMed]
15. Sowder, A.M.; Witt, B.L.; Hunt, J.P. An update on the risk of lymph node metastasis for the follicular variant of papillary thyroid carcinoma with the new diagnostic paradigm. *Head Neck Pathol.* **2018**, *12*, 105–109. [CrossRef] [PubMed]
16. Schmidt, R.L.; Jedrzkiewicz, J.D.; Allred, R.J.; Matsuoka, S.; Witt, B.L. Verification bias in diagnostic accuracy studies for fine- and core needle biopsy of salivary gland lesions in otolaryngology journals: A systematic review and analysis. *Head Neck* **2014**, *36*, 1654–1661. [CrossRef] [PubMed]
17. Huyett, P.; Monaco, S.E.; Choi, S.S.; Simons, J.P. Utility of fine-needle aspiration biopsy in the evaluation of pediatric head and neck masses. *Otolaryngol. Head Neck Surg.* **2016**, *154*, 928–935. [CrossRef] [PubMed]
18. Cibas, E.S.; Ducatman, B.S. *Cytology. Diagnostic Principles and Clinical Correlates*; Saunders, Elsevier: Philadelphia, PA, USA, 2009.
19. Demay, R.M. *The Art & Science of Cytopathology*, 2nd ed.; American Society for Clinical Pathology: Chicago, IL, USA, 2011; Volume 4.
20. Jain, M.; Majumdar, D.D.; Agarwal, K.; Bais, A.S.; Choudhury, M. FNAC as a diagnostic tool in pediatric head and neck lesions. *Indian Pediatr.* **1999**, *36*, 921–923. [PubMed]
21. Mittra, P.; Bharti, R.; Pandey, M.K. Role of fine needle aspiration cytology in head and neck lesions of paediatric age group. *J. Clin. Diagn. Res.* **2013**, *7*, 1055–1058. [CrossRef] [PubMed]
22. Shirian, S.; Daneshbod, Y.; Haghpanah, S.; Khademi, B.; Noorbakhsh, F.; Ghaemi, A.; Mosayebi, Z. Spectrum of pediatric tumors diagnosed by fine-needle aspiration cytology. *Medicine* **2017**, *96*, e5480. [CrossRef] [PubMed]
23. Ellies, M.; Laskawi, R. Diseases of the salivary glands in infants and adolescents. *Head Face Med.* **2010**, *6*, 1. [CrossRef] [PubMed]
24. Rutt, A.L.; Hawkshaw, M.J.; Lurie, D.; Sataloff, R.T. Salivary gland cancer in patients younger than 30 years. *Ear Nose Throat J.* **2011**, *90*, 174–184. [PubMed]
25. Iro, H.; Zenk, J. Salivary gland diseases in children. *GMS Curr. Top. Otorhinolaryngol. Head Neck Surg.* **2014**, *13*, Doc06. [CrossRef] [PubMed]
26. Colella, G.; Cannavale, R.; Flamminio, F.; Foschini, M.P. Fine-needle aspiration cytology of salivary gland lesions: A systematic review. *J. Oral Maxillofac. Surg.* **2010**, *68*, 2146–2153. [CrossRef] [PubMed]

27. Eneroth, C.M. Incidence and prognosis of salivary-gland tumours at different sites. A study of parotid, submandibular and palatal tumours in 2632 patients. *Acta Otolaryngol. Suppl.* **1969**, *263*, 174–178. [CrossRef] [PubMed]

28. Lewis, A.G.; Tong, T.; Maghami, E. Diagnosis and management of malignant salivary gland tumors of the parotid gland. *Otolaryngol. Clin. N. Am.* **2016**, *49*, 343–380. [CrossRef] [PubMed]

29. Wojtczak, B.; Sutkowski, K.; Glod, M.; Czopnik, P.; Rzeszutko, M.; Jawiarczyk-Przybylowska, A.; Bolanowski, M. Neck nodular lesions mimicking thyroid tumors. *Neuro Endocrinol. Lett.* **2013**, *34*, 606–609. [PubMed]

30. Goonewardene, S.A.; Nasuti, J.F. Value of mucin detection in distinguishing mucoepidermoid carcinoma from warthin's tumor on fine needle aspiration. *Acta Cytol.* **2002**, *46*, 704–708. [CrossRef] [PubMed]

31. Griffith, C.C.; Schmitt, A.C.; Pantanowitz, L.; Monaco, S.E. A pattern-based risk-stratification scheme for salivary gland cytology: A multi-institutional, interobserver variability study to determine applicability. *Cancer Cytopathol.* **2017**, *125*, 776–785. [CrossRef] [PubMed]

32. Pantanowitz, L.; Thompson, L.D.R.; Rossi, E.D. Diagnostic approach to fine needle aspirations of cystic lesions of the salivary gland. *Head Neck Pathol.* **2018**. [CrossRef] [PubMed]

33. Rohilla, M.; Gupta, N.; Singh, P.; Rajwanshi, A. Reply to application of the milan system for reporting risk stratification in salivary gland cytopathology. *Cancer Cytopathol.* **2018**, *126*, 71. [CrossRef] [PubMed]

34. Rohilla, M.; Singh, P.; Rajwanshi, A.; Gupta, N.; Srinivasan, R.; Dey, P.; Vashishta, R.K. Three-year cytohistological correlation of salivary gland FNA cytology at a tertiary center with the application of the milan system for risk stratification. *Cancer Cytopathol.* **2017**, *125*, 767–775. [CrossRef] [PubMed]

35. Rossi, E.D.; Faquin, W.C.; Baloch, Z.; Barkan, G.A.; Foschini, M.P.; Pusztaszeri, M.; Vielh, P.; Kurtycz, D.F.I. The milan system for reporting salivary gland cytopathology: Analysis and suggestions of initial survey. *Cancer Cytopathol.* **2017**, *125*, 757–766. [CrossRef] [PubMed]

36. Pusztaszeri, M.; Baloch, Z.; Vielh, P.; Faquin, W.C. Application of the Milan system for reporting risk stratification in salivary gland cytopathology. *Cancer Cytopathol.* **2018**, *126*, 69–70. [CrossRef] [PubMed]

37. Rapkiewicz, A.; Thuy Le, B.; Simsir, A.; Cangiarella, J.; Levine, P. Spectrum of head and neck lesions diagnosed by fine-needle aspiration cytology in the pediatric population. *Cancer* **2007**, *111*, 242–251. [CrossRef] [PubMed]

38. Handa, U.; Mohan, H.; Bal, A. Role of fine needle aspiration cytology in evaluation of paediatric lymphadenopathy. *Cytopathology* **2003**, *14*, 66–69. [CrossRef] [PubMed]

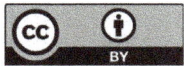

diagnostics

MDPI

Article

Preterm Perinatal Hypoxia-Ischemia Does not Affect Somatosensory Evoked Potentials in Adult Rats

Melinda Barkhuizen [1,2,3,†], Johan S.H. Vles [2,4,†], Ralph van Mechelen [1,2], Marijne Vermeer [1,2], Boris W. Kramer [1,2], Peter Chedraui [5], Paul Bergs [6], Vivianne H.J.M. van Kranen-Mastenbroek [6] and Antonio W.D. Gavilanes [1,2,5,*]

[1] Department of Pediatrics, Maastricht University Medical Centre (MUMC), 6229HX, Maastricht, The Netherlands; m.barkhuizen@maastrichtuniversity.nl (M.B.); r.vanmechelen@maastrichtuniversity.nl (R.v.M.); marijne.vermeer@gmail.com (M.V.); b.kramer@mumc.nl (B.W.K.)

[2] Department of Translational Neuroscience, School for Mental Health and Neuroscience (MHeNs), Maastricht University, 6229 HX, Maastricht, The Netherlands; jsh.vles@mumc.nl

[3] DST/NWU Preclinical Drug Development Platform, North-West University, Potchefstroom 2531, South Africa

[4] Child Neurology, Maastricht University Medical Centre, 6229 HX, Maastricht, The Netherlands

[5] Instituto de Investigación e Innovación de Salud Integral, Facultad de Ciencias Médicas, Universidad Católica de Santiago de Guayaquil, Guayaquil 090615, Ecuador; peterchedraui@yahoo.com

[6] Clinical Neurophysiology, Maastricht University Medical Centre, 6229 HX Maastricht, The Netherlands; p.bergs@mumc.nl (P.B.); v.kranen.mastenbroek@mumc.nl (V.H.J.M.v.K.-M.)

* Correspondence: danilo.gavilanes@mumc.nl; Tel.: +31-433876061

† These authors contributed equally to this work.

Received: 16 August 2019; Accepted: 12 September 2019; Published: 18 September 2019

Abstract: Somatosensory evoked potentials (SSEPs) are a valuable tool to assess functional integrity of the somatosensory pathways and for the prediction of sensorimotor outcome in perinatal injuries, such as perinatal hypoxia-ischemia (HI). In the present research, we studied the translational potential of SSEPs together with sensory function in the male adult rat with perinatal HI compared to the male healthy adult rat. Both somatosensory response and evoked potential were measured at 10-11 months after global perinatal HI. Clear evoked potentials were obtained, but there were no group differences in the amplitude or latency of the evoked potentials of the preceding sensory response. The bilateral tactile stimulation test was also normal in both groups. This lack of effect may be ascribed to the late age-of-testing and functional recovery of the rats.

Keywords: somatosensory evoked potential; preterm brain; rat model; cerebral palsy; hypoxia-ischemia

1. Introduction

Somatosensory evoked potentials (SSEPs) are a valuable tool to assess functional integrity of the somatosensory pathways of the peripheral and central nervous systems [1]. SSEPs are widely used for the prediction of motor outcomes in perinatal injuries, where the long-term effects of the injury are difficult to ascertain early in life [2]. Hypoxic-ischemic encephalopathy (HIE) is a common injury in neonates, with a global occurrence of 8.5 infants per 1000 live births in 2010 [3]. Infants with HIE, especially preterm infants, are considered to be at risk for developmental disorders [4]. They present a heterogeneous clinical picture, varying by individual, and ranging from major disorders like cerebral palsy (CP) to less severe impairments like developmental coordination disorder (DCD). DCD is commonly associated with other developmental comorbidities, including attention deficit/hyperactivity disorder (ADHD) and learning disabilities, and could be related to an impaired sensory process.

Several studies have shown that SSEPs, in combination with other electrophysiological tools and neuroimaging, are useful in the diagnosis of encephalopathy after HIE and could improve the prediction of infants that will have poor neurodevelopment outcomes two years after perinatal HIE [2,5–7]. However, the predictive value of SSEPs decreases with longer follow-up periods. Neonatal SSEP latencies do not correlate with neurodevelopmental outcomes at school-going age in infants with mild HIE. The long-term prognostic value of neonatal SSEPs in this patient group is unclear [1]. It is also unknown whether the neonatal SSEP abnormalities persist in adults with HIE. On the other hand, SSEPs are suited to evaluate patients suffering from more severe forms of disability such as cerebral palsy (CP), in whom neurological deficits might reflect disruption of motor as well as sensory connections [8,9], suggesting a neural network disorder. Furthermore, both motor and behavioral skills involve the process of receiving a sensory input. In this context, motor-behavioral deficits could be treated by sensory-based therapies. Indeed, this may be acceptable as one component of a comprehensive treatment plan in the management of children with developmental, behavioral, and motor disorders of different etiology [10].

SSEP is a relatively simple, objective, and reproducible diagnostic procedure that assesses the effect of the somatosensory input in the peripheral and central neuronal networks. In the present experiments, we used a perinatal rat model of hypoxic-ischemia (HI) injury by submersion [11]. Previous studies using this model of global perinatal preterm HI demonstrated that severe HI (submersion lasting for 19–20 min) decreased locomotor activity in the adult rat, while milder HI insults might increase locomotion [12,13]. In this respect, our experimental group is a cohort of male adult rats that recovered from moderate global perinatal HI and showed cognitive (memory) as well as motor abnormalities (hyperactivity) within the spectrum of ADHD at the age of 6–8 months [14]. To test whether this cohort had a problem in coordination (DCD), we evaluated the sensory functioning using a bilateral tactile stimulation test and we recorded cortical SSEPs after unilateral tibial nerve stimulation at 11 months of age [14].

The present study reports the outcomes of the SSEPs and behavioral tasks of sensory functioning of male adult rats subjected to moderate perinatal HI. We hypothesized that long-term sensory deficits were relevant to the combined sensory and motor deficits previously demonstrated in this cohort of male rats after perinatal HI.

2. Materials and Methods

2.1. Rodents and Ethics Approval

The experiments were performed in Sprague-Dawley rats from Charles River (Leiden, The Netherlands). The rats were housed at the Central Animal Experimentation Facilities of the Maastricht University, The Netherlands. Experimental female rats were synchronized with luteinizing hormone-releasing hormone (Cat. L4513, Sigma-Aldrich, The Netherlands), and time-mated between 15:00 and 07:00 the following morning. All experiments were conducted under ethical approval from the Dutch Central Committee for Animal Testing according to the guidelines of the EU directive 2010/63/EU (approval code: AVD107002016540, approved on 16 July 2016).

2.2. Perinatal Hypoxia-Ischemia (HI) Procedure

In the afternoon of embryonic day 21 (expected delivery on E21–E22), a pregnant female rat was euthanized by rapid decapitation and the uterine horns, still containing the pups, rapidly removed and submerged in saline solution at 37 °C for 16–18 min according to previously-described methodology [12,13]. After submersion, the pups were delivered, manually stimulated to breathe, and placed in a closed pediatric incubator to recover for an hour (HI group). The control Cesarean-section rats (C-section) were delivered from the same litters without submersion and placed in the closed pediatric incubator to recover with their HI littermates. After recovery, the mixed litter of HI and C-section pups was placed with a foster mother that had given birth the day before to minimize the impact of maternal care differences on outcomes. The mortality rate for the HI procedure was 39%.

2.3. Housing

After weaning, the rats were fed a standard laboratory diet and housed in pairs in individually ventilated cages, up to 8 months of age, when they were housed 4 per cage in larger filter top cages. The rats were housed on a reverse day night cycle (lights off at 7:00/lights on at 19:00).

2.4. Adhesive Removal ('Sticker Test')

The adhesive removal test was performed at 10 months of age. Somatosensory response was assessed with a bilateral tactile stimulation test adapted from a method previously reported [15,16]. For the sticker test, rats were placed in an empty cage with videotaping from the sides. One investigator restrained the rat, whilst another investigator placed two brightly colored circular adhesive labels (1.27 cm diameter, Avery office products, Houten, The Netherlands) on the dorsum of both forepaws of the rat. Adult rats normally touch and remove the stickers with their teeth. The time from placing the rat in the arena to the initial purposeful sticker contact ('noticed') and to removal from both paws ('removed') was recorded and the latency time from initial contact to removal was calculated. The time limit for adhesive removal was 180 s. Group sizes for this test were C-section ($n = 12$) and HI ($n = 11$).

2.5. Sedation

For the SSEPs, the rats were placed under anesthesia with an induction of midazolam (0.5 mg/kg), followed by a mixture of ketamine (0.75 mg/kg), medetomidine (0.06 mg/kg) and atropine (0.04 mg/kg) in saline (KMA). Sedation was maintained during the procedure with an intraperitoneal infusion of the KMA mixture.

2.6. Somatosensory Evoked Potentials (SSEPs)

The SSEP was conducted according to methodology previously described by Zhang, et al. [17] at the age of 11 months. A Nicolet Viking IV P™ (Nicolet Biomedical, Madison, WI, USA) was utilized to record and analyze the waveform of SSEPs. Twelve-millimeter long monopolar needle electrodes with attached lead wire were used for active, reference, and ground electrodes. A sedated rat was placed on a board and the needle electrodes were carefully inserted into the scalp and placed on the surface of the skull, parallel with the long axis of the rat body. The active electrode was located on the midline of the skull and crossed the point of bregma for right hemisphere recording.

The reference electrode was placed on the skull surface over the olfactory bulb and the ground electrode was placed in the shoulder. Left tibial nerve stimulation was performed with 0.2 ms pulses at 1.7 Hz (filter set to 2–3000 Hz) with an intensity of 1–3 mA, depending on the twitch response, for an average of 500 stimuli. We studied the cortical SSEPs P_1 and N_2 amplitudes and latencies, which were registered by a child neurologist (JSHV) and reviewed together with a clinical neurophysiologist (VHvKM) and a clinical neurophysiology technician (PB).

We recorded 6 male rats per group, for the following groups: C-section (body weights: 601 ± 36 g) and HI (body weights: 574 ± 33 g).

2.7. Statistics

Stata 10 (Statacorp, TX, USA) was used to assess group differences by means of the non-parametric Kruskal-Wallis H-test followed by post-hoc Dunn's test of equality. Regarding SSEPs, the averaged value between two runs was used. *P* values <0.05 were considered as statistically significant. Figures regarding average ± standard error means were constructed with GraphPad Prism 6 (GraphPad Software Inc., La Jolla, CA, USA). Outliers were not considered in the analysis.

3. Results

3.1. Adhesive Removal Test ('Sticker Test')

The results of the sticker test are shown in Figure 1. There were no significant differences between groups regarding the time the rats took to notice the sticker on their paws ($p = 0.943$), the time to remove it ($p = 0.546$), or the time from notice to removal ($p = 0.244$).

Sticker removal test

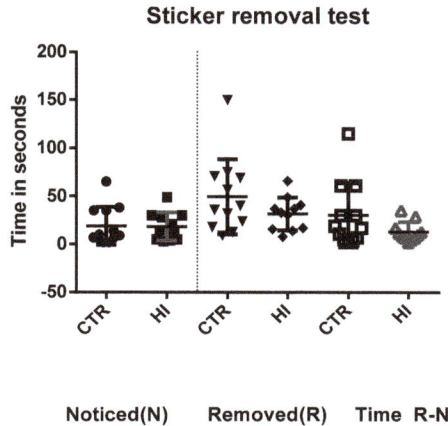

Noticed(N)   Removed(R)   Time R-N

Figure 1. The adhesive removal test showing the latency to notice (N) and remove the stickers from the front paws (R), as well as the time elapsed between notice and removal (R-N). CTR: control C-section group, HI: hypoxia-ischemia group.

3.2. Evoked Potentials

Reproducible SSEPs were obtained in all rats. After exclusion of one outlier, our group sizes were: C-section ($n = 5$) and HI ($n = 6$). There were no significant differences for the amplitude of the P_1 peak ($p = 0.078$), the N_2 peak ($p = 0.891$), or the absolute difference in the amplitude of the P_1-N_2 peaks ($p = 0.469$). There were also no significant group effects on the latencies of these peaks P_1 ($p = 0.667$), N_2 ($p = 0.558$) (Figures 2 and 3). Exclusion of the outlier did not statistically change the results.

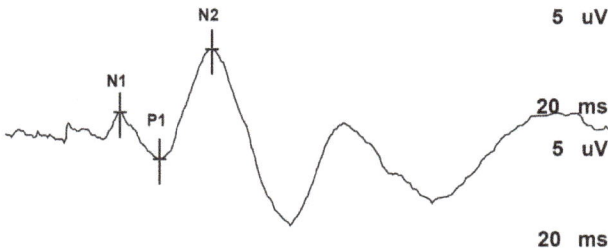

Figure 2. Representative example of tibial somatosensory evoked potentials (SSEPs) recording in adult rats. N_1, P_1 and N_2 cortical latency and amplitude.

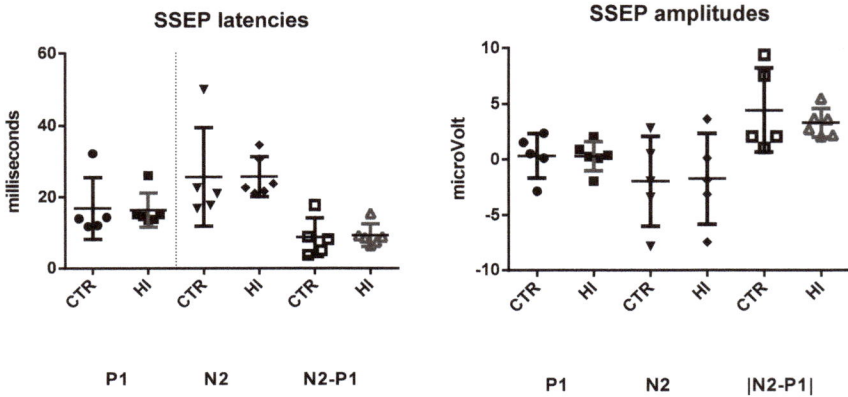

Figure 3. The latencies and amplitudes of the SSEP test. Each data point represents a single male animal; horizontal lines represent regional medians with the standard error medians. P1 latencies, N2 latencies, P1 amplitude, N2 amplitude, Absolute differences in amplitude. CTR: control C-section group, HI: hypoxia-ischemia group.

4. Discussion

In human newborns, particularly those born preterm, HI is an important cause of long-term neurological disabilities, such as learning and memory deficits and sensorimotor and motor functioning deficits like CP [18,19]. The present study investigated the long-term effects of moderate HI on somatosensory functioning in male survivors using an established rat model of preterm HI.

Recording of SSEPs is a quantitative method for evaluation of both the central and peripheral nervous system. Peripheral sensory information reaches the parietal-occipital cortex by thalamocortical pathways e.g., corona radiata and internal capsule. The parietal cortex connects to neocortical areas including premotor, prefrontal areas as well as to the cerebellum through pontine nuclei. Merging this information with the basal ganglia, pre-Rolandic motor areas control motor activity through the descending corticospinal tracts [20]. SSEPs are suited to evaluate children and adult patients suffering from CP [9]. Through the findings of neuroimaging studies, a correlation has been reported in CP patients between disrupted descending corticospinal pathways and disrupted thalamocortical pathways connecting to the sensory cortex [20]. The role of SSEPs in children and adults with milder deficits after HI is unclear. Identifiable sensory processing and motor interaction during early childhood, e.g., reaching and touching objects using hands and mouth, provides a critical foundation for normal growth, development, and learning. This sensorimotor integration explains why sensory impairments affect motor recovery, and why sensory based strategies might promote motor and behavioral recovery.

The seminal work reported by de Louw, et al. (2002) on the short-term effect of severe perinatal HI on spinal cord apoptosis using this perinatal model of submersion showed an increased lumbar grey and white-matter apoptosis [21]. These changes may contribute to the permanent motor deficits, which are the main neurological manifestations of brain injury in the premature infant. We investigated whether preterm HI had a long-term effect on expected sensorimotor deficits.

In the adhesive removal test, we did not observe a statistically significant effect of HI. We used the time for removal from both paws, since we caused a global insult which was expected to affect both hemispheres equally. In adult rats with unilateral lesions, a bias to touching the non-affected forepaw first has been reported [15]. A previous study of neonatal unilateral hypoxic-ischemic injury also did not find significant group differences with the adhesive removal among five-week-old rats with a modest brain injury [16].

Tibial SSEPs evaluate the somatosensory pathway including dorsal columns of the rat's spinal cord and the contralateral parietal cortex. Our study found that the perinatal HI insult did not influence the SSEPs. A previous study with SSEPs after neonatal stroke in the rat, found profound unilateral changes in SSEPs one week after the insult, but recovery of the deficits 3 weeks postnatally. This may indicate large-scale plasticity of the somatosensory networks even after a unilateral neonatal injury [22]. It is thus possible that sufficient recovery occurred at 11 months after the global asphyxic insult and ameliorated changes observed in evoked potentials.

SSEPs were performed unilaterally (left tibialis nerve stimulation) assuming symmetrical and global central nervous system impact inherent to the global perinatal hypoxic-ischemic insult. This statement has been corroborated by the symmetrical adhesive removal test, which complements the SSEP data. In summary, we did not find any permanent significant sensory behavioral or electrophysiological changes in rat adulthood explaining the hyperactivity disorder and recognition memory deficit shown by this rat cohort. However, these results raise the question whether the somatosensory functioning of our rats has sufficiently recovered over time, or whether the SSEPs was not sensitive enough to detect deficits in adult rats.

There are several methodological and study limitations that could explain why we failed to detect preclinical SSEPs:

(a) Due to our cross-sectional design, we might have missed SSEP changes in early postnatal age and adolescence.

(b) Midazolam, ketamine and medetomidine were used as systemic anesthetics during SSEPs recordings. Accordingly, this anesthetic combination may have influenced SSEPs results; however, both experimental groups received the same anesthetic regime [23]. In humans, SSEPs are known to be less sensitive to the injectable anesthetics that we used, than to inhalation anesthetics [24].

(c) The lumbar spinal cord apoptosis observed in severe HI models (19–20 min of submersion) may not necessarily be the postnatal hallmark of the moderate HI model (16–18 min of submersion) used in this experiment [21].

(d) Evidence supports more neurological impairments and higher mortality for male preterm infants. In line with the human data, behavioral studies have consistently shown that the male sex is associated with an increased risk of long-term motor deficits in the rat preterm HIE [11]. Therefore, only male rats were included in this study.

(e) Our global HI insult was conducted around the time of birth, when the rodent brain development is comparable to that of human infants born at a very low gestational age [11]. Studying SSEPs in larger animal models with brain development comparable to humans, such as sheep, may be more predictive of the human clinical situation [25]. However, larger animals are less suitable for chronic, long term studies.

Despite the aforementioned limitations, the present study found that, in the rat, moderate global HI did not influence the sensorimotor measurements assessed at 11 months. The moderate severity of the insult and the neuroplasticity observed early in life may explain the lack of a measurable effect on the adult survivors. More research is warranted to further confirm our results.

Highlights:

1. SSEPs are used to clinically assess the integrity of peripheral and central somatosensory pathways after perinatal HI.

2. Childhood SSEPs are often used to predict long-term outcomes, but it is unknown if sensory pathway deficits persist into adulthood.

3. We showed the electrophysiological and behavioral integrity of the somatosensory pathways in adult rats subjected to moderate perinatal HI.

Author Contributions: M.B., R.v.M., M.V.: Conducted the HI experiments when the rats were born. M.B., R.v.M., J.S.H.V.: Conducted SSEP measurements and adhesive removal test. P.B., V.H.J.M.v.K.-M.: Interpreted SSEP measurements. B.W.K., P.C., A.W.D.G., J.S.H.V.: Conceptualized experiments and provided global supervision. M.B., J.S.H.V., A.W.D.G.: Wrote first draft. All authors: Commented on drafts, approved final drafts.

Funding: This research was partially supported by the Sistema de Investigación y Desarrollo (SINDE) of the Universidad Católica de Santiago de Guayaquil, Guayaquil, Ecuador, through the grant No SIU- 319: Perinatal asphyxia and stem cell treatment. M. Barkhuizen is funded by the National Research Foundation of South Africa (Grant specific reference number 89230 and 98217) and the Foundation of Paediatrics, Maastricht University Medical Centre +. All views expressed in this article are those of the authors and not of the funding agencies.

Conflicts of Interest: The authors declare no conflict of interest.

Abbreviations

CP	cerebral palsy
HI	hypoxia ischemia
SSEPs	somatosensory evoked potentials
HIE	hypoxic ischemic encephalopathy
ADHD	attention deficit/hyperactivity disorder
DCD	developmental coordination disorder

References

1. Trollmann, R.; Nüsken, E.; Wenzel, D. Neonatal Somatosensory Evoked Potentials: Maturational Aspects and Prognostic Value. *Pediatr. Neurol.* **2010**, *42*, 427–433. [CrossRef]

2. Swarte, R.M.; Cherian, P.J.; Lequin, M.; Visser, G.H.; Govaert, P. Somatosensory evoked potentials are of additional prognostic value in certain patterns of brain injury in term birth asphyxia. *Clin. Neurophysiol.* **2012**, *123*, 1631–1638. [CrossRef]

3. Lee, A.C.; Kozuki, N.; Blencowe, H.; Vos, T.; Bahalim, A.; Darmstadt, G.L.; Niermeyer, S.; Ellis, M.; Robertson, N.J.; Cousens, S.; et al. Intrapartum-related neonatal encephalopathy incidence and impairment at regional and global levels for 2010 with trends from 1990. *Pediatr. Res.* **2013**, *74*, 50–72. [CrossRef]

4. Volpe, J.J. The neurological outcome of perinatal asphyxia. In *Early Brain Damage V1: Research Orientations and Clinical Observations*; Academic Press: Cambridge, MA, USA, 2012; p. 151.

5. Nevalainen, P.; Marchi, V.; Metsäranta, M.; Lönnqvist, T.; Toiviainen-Salo, S.; Vanhatalo, S.; Lauronen, L. Evoked potentials recorded during routine EEG predict outcome after perinatal asphyxia. *Clin. Neurophysiol.* **2017**, *128*, 1337–1343. [CrossRef]

6. Garfinkle, J.; Sant'Anna, G.M.; Rosenblatt, B.; Majnemer, A.; Wintermark, P.; Shevell, M.I. Somatosensory evoked potentials in neonates with hypoxic-ischemic encephalopathy treated with hypothermia. *Eur. J. Paediatr. Neurol.* **2015**, *19*, 423–428. [CrossRef]

7. Suppiej, A.; Cappellari, A.; Franzoi, M.; Traverso, A.; Ermani, M.; Zanardo, V. Bilateral loss of cortical somatosensory evoked potential at birth predicts cerebral palsy in term and near-term newborns. *Early Hum. Dev.* **2010**, *86*, 93–98. [CrossRef]

8. Riquelme, I.; Montoya, P. Developmental changes in somatosensory processing in cerebral palsy and healthy individuals. *Clin. Neurophysiol.* **2010**, *121*, 1314–1320. [CrossRef]

9. Teflioudi, E.P.; Zafeiriou, D.I.; Vargiami, E.; Kontopoulos, E.; Tsikoulas, I. Somatosensory Evoked Potentials in Children With Bilateral Spastic Cerebral Palsy. *Pediatr. Neurol.* **2011**, *44*, 177–182. [CrossRef]

10. Zimmer, M.; Desch, L. Sensory Integration Therapies for Children with Developmental and Behavioral Disorders. *Pediatrics* **2012**, *129*, 1186–1189.

11. Barkhuizen, M.; Hove, D.V.D.; Vles, J.; Steinbusch, H.; Kramer, B.; Gavilanes, A. 25 years of research on global asphyxia in the immature rat brain. *Neurosci. Biobehav. Rev.* **2017**, *75*, 166–182. [CrossRef]

12. Strackx, E.; Hove, D.L.V.D.; Prickaerts, J.; Zimmermann, L.; Steinbusch, H.W.; Blanco, C.E.; Gavilanes, A.D.; Vles, J.H.; Gavilanes, A.W. Fetal asphyctic preconditioning protects against perinatal asphyxia-induced behavioral consequences in adulthood. *Behav. Brain Res.* **2010**, *208*, 343–351. [CrossRef]

13. Loidl, C.; Gavilanes, A.; Van Dijk, E.H.; Vreuls, W.; Blokland, A.; Vles, J.S.; Steinbusch, H.W.; Blanco, C.E.; Gavilanes, A.W. Effects of hypothermia and gender on survival and behavior after perinatal asphyxia in rats. *Physiol. Behav.* **2000**, *68*, 263–269. [CrossRef]

14. Barkhuizen, M.; Van Mechelen, R.; Vermeer, M.; Chedraui, P.; Paes, D.; Hove, D.L.V.D.; Vaes, B.; Mays, R.W.; Steinbusch, H.W.; Robertson, N.J.; et al. Systemic multipotent adult progenitor cells improve long-term neurodevelopmental outcomes after preterm hypoxic-ischemic encephalopathy. *Behav. Brain Res.* **2019**, *362*, 77–81. [CrossRef]

15. Schallert, T.; Fleming, S.M.; Leasure, J.L.; Tillerson, J.L.; Bland, S.T. CNS plasticity and assessment of forelimb sensorimotor outcome in unilateral rat models of stroke, cortical ablation, parkinsonism and spinal cord injury. *Neuropharmacology* **2000**, *39*, 777–787. [CrossRef]

16. Grow, J.L.; Liu, Y.Q.; Barks, J.D. Can Lateralizing Sensorimotor Deficits Be Identified after Neonatal Cerebral Hypoxia-Ischemia in Rats? *Dev. Neurosci.* **2003**, *25*, 394–402. [CrossRef]

17. Zhang, S.-X.; Huang, F.; Gates, M.; Holmberg, E.G. Somatosensory evoked potentials can be recorded on the midline of the skull with subdermal electrodes in non-sedated rats elicited by magnetic stimulation of the tibial nerve. *J. Neurosci. Methods* **2012**, *208*, 114–118. [CrossRef]

18. Braddick, O.; Atkinson, J.; Innocenti, G. Perinatal brain damage in children: Neuroplasticity, early intervention, and molecular mechanisms of recovery. In *Gene Expression to Neurobiology and Behaviour: Human Brain Development and Developmental Disorders*; Elsevier: Amsterdam, The Netherlands, 2011; Volume 189, p. 139.

19. Van Handel, M.; Swaab, H.; De Vries, L.S.; Jongmans, M.J. Long-term cognitive and behavioral consequences of neonatal encephalopathy following perinatal asphyxia: A review. *Eur. J. Nucl. Med. Mol. Imaging* **2007**, *166*, 645–654. [CrossRef]

20. Hoon, A.H., Jr.; Stashinko, E.E.; Nagae, L.M.; Lin, D.D.; Keller, J.; Bastian, A.; Campbell, M.L.; Levey, E.; Mori, S.; Johnston, M.V. Sensory and motor deficits in children with cerebral palsy born preterm correlate with diffusion tensor imaging abnormalities in thalamocortical pathways. *Dev. Med. Child Neurol.* **2009**, *51*, 697–704. [CrossRef]

21. De Louw, A.; De Vente, J.; Steinbusch, H.; Gavilanes, A.W.; Steinbusch, H.; Blanco, C.; Troost, J.; Vles, J. Apoptosis in the rat spinal cord during postnatal development; the effect of perinatal asphyxia on programmed cell death. *Neuroscience* **2002**, *112*, 751–758. [CrossRef]

22. Quairiaux, C.; Sizonenko, S.V.; Mégevand, P.; Michel, C.M.; Kiss, J.Z. Functional Deficit and Recovery of Developing Sensorimotor Networks following Neonatal Hypoxic-Ischemic Injury in the Rat. *Cereb. Cortex* **2010**, *20*, 2080–2091. [CrossRef]

23. Hayton, S.M.; Kriss, A.; Muller, D.P. Comparison of the effects of four anaesthetic agents on somatosensory evoked potentials in the rat. *Lab Anim.* **1999**, *33*, 243–251. [CrossRef]

24. Becker, A.; Amlong, C.; Rusy, D.A. Somatosensory-Evoked Potentials. In *Monitoring the Nervous System for Anesthesiologists and Other Health Care Professionals*; Springer International Publishing AG: Cham, Switzerland, 2017; pp. 3–18.

25. Anegroaie, P.; Frasch, M.; Rupprecht, S.; Antonow-Schlorke, I.; Müller, T.; Schubert, H.; Witte, O.; Schwab, M. Development of somatosensory-evoked potentials in foetal sheep: Effects of betamethasone. *Acta Physiol.* **2017**, *220*, 137–149. [CrossRef]

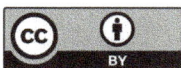

diagnostics

MDPI

Review

Clinicopathological Spectrum of Bilirubin Encephalopathy/Kernicterus

Sumit Das [1,2,*] and Frank K.H. van Landeghem [1,2]

[1] Division of Neuropathology, University of Alberta and Stollery Children's Hospital, Edmonton, AB T6G 2B7, Canada; vanlande@ualberta.ca

[2] Neuroscience and Mental Health Institute, University of Alberta, Edmonton, AB T6G 2B7, Canada

* Correspondence: sumit1@ualberta.ca; Tel.: +01-780-407-7205

Received: 2 February 2019; Accepted: 25 February 2019; Published: 28 February 2019

Abstract: Bilirubin encephalopathy/kernicterus is relatively rare, but continues to occur despite universal newborn screening. What is more interesting is the spectrum of clinical and even neuropathological findings that have been reported in the literature to be associated with bilirubin encephalopathy and kernicterus. In this review, the authors discuss the array of clinicopathological findings reported in the context of bilirubin encephalopathy and kernicterus, as well as the types of diagnostic testing used in patients suspected of having bilirubin encephalopathy or kernicterus. The authors aim to raise the awareness of these features among both pediatric neurologists and neuropathologists.

Keywords: bilirubin encephalopathy; kernicterus; neurological symptoms; diagnosis; neuropathology

1. Introduction

Bilirubin encephalopathy/kernicterus is a relatively uncommon occurrence. Although neonatal jaundice is quite common, affecting 60%–80% of newborns overall [1], severe hyperbilirubinemia (> 20 mg/dL) that could potentially lead to kernicterus and neurodevelopmental complications is said to be much rarer, affecting less than 2% of newborn infants [2]. Associated risk factors can include a low gestational age, low birth weight, hemolysis, sepsis, cephalohematoma or easy bruising, and exclusive breast feeding. Recent literature has shed light on the wide range of clinical symptomology and pathological findings associated with bilirubin encephalopathy/kernicterus [3,4]. Bilirubin-induced neurological complications continue to occur in industrialized countries, but a disproportionately increased burden is reported in low- and middle-income countries, primarily because of delays in delivering treatments that are more readily available in high-income countries [1,5]. This review aims to provide a comprehensive overview of the clinical, radiological, and neuropathological features associated with bilirubin encephalopathy/kernicterus that have been reported in the literature, as well as the string of diagnostic tests used in patients suspected of having bilirubin encephalopathy or kernicterus. The authors hope to raise awareness of the wide spectrum of findings that should raise the possibility of bilirubin encephalopathy or kernicterus to pediatric neurologists and neuropathologists alike.

2. Clinical Presentation

Acute bilirubin encephalopathy encompasses the acute illness caused by severe hyperbilirubinemia. Presenting signs and symptoms include decreased feeding, lethargy, abnormal tone (hypotonia and/or hypertonia), high-pitched cry, retrocollis and opisthotonus, setting-sun sign, fever, seizures, and possibly death [6,7]. Seizures usually resolve several weeks after the acute insult. Therefore, persistent seizures in a child with kernicterus should prompt a search for another concomitant condition.

The so-called 'kernicteric facies' in acute bilirubin encephalopathy includes a combination of the setting-sun sign (i.e., paresis of upward gaze) with eyelid retraction, which together comprise the Collier sign, and facial dystonia. These findings make the infant appear stunned, scared, or anxious. Some infants may also exhibit disconjugate or wondering eyes. This kernicteric facies persists for at least two to three weeks after acute bilirubin encephalopathy [8].

Recent reviews and studies have also reported apnea in both preterm and term infants in conjunction with other findings of acute bilirubin encephalopathy and also as an isolated early abnormality [9–11]. Apnea may also be a sign of seizures in a newborn with jaundice, albeit infrequently. These authors also suggested that apneic events are a common clinical sign of bilirubin neurotoxicity in late preterm and term neonates with severe jaundice associated with bilirubin levels greater than 25 mg/dL. Clinical findings suggestive of bilirubin-induced disturbance in control of breathing include (1) new onset of frequent apnea, bradycardia, and desaturations concurrent with marked hyperbilirubinemia; (2) apnea, bradycardia, and desaturation that require intubation and assisted ventilation in an infant with marked hyperbilirubinemia; and (3) acute worsening of frequency and severity of apnea from baseline levels in an infant with marked hyperbilirubinemia [9]. Any noticeable change in the frequency and/or severity of apnea should prompt a measurement of total serum bilirubin levels as it may suggest acute bilirubin encephalopathy.

Kernicterus describes the long-term outcome of acute bilirubin encephalopathy and encompasses a tetrad of clinical features that are typically evident after one year of age: (i) abnormal motor control, movements, and muscle tone; (ii) an auditory processing disturbance with or without hearing loss; (iii) oculomotor impairments, especially impairment of the upward vertical gaze; and (iv) dysplasia of the enamel of deciduous (baby) teeth [12].

Auditory complications, a disabling neurological finding in kernicterus, are typically characterized by varying degrees of auditory neuropathy/dys-synchrony (AN/AD) ranging from central auditory processing difficulties with normal hearing to severe AN/AD with absent auditory brainstem responses, and possibly accompanying severe hearing loss and deafness [12]. In fact, the brainstem cochlear nuclei are said to be one of the first structures affected by elevated total bilirubin, followed by the auditory nerve [13,14]. Although the cochlea is not directly affected by elevated bilirubin levels, it is thought that damage to the cochlea may occur secondary to damage to the cochlear nucleus and/or auditory nerve [15].

Patients with so-called 'motor predominant' kernicterus due to lesions in the globus pallidus (interna and externa) and subthalamic nucleus reportedly present with an athetotic or dyskinetic form of cerebral palsy. In the most severe form of 'motor predominant' kernicterus, one may observe severe dystonia/athetosis that prevents voluntary movements, including ambulation, speech, and self-feeding, and may be accompanied by severe hypertonia and muscle cramping. Mild and moderate forms of kernicterus may also present with motor symptoms that include dystonia with or without athetosis and gross motor developmental delays, although patients with moderate kernicterus may experience greater difficulty ambulating due to choreoathetoid movements [16].

Bilirubin-induced neurological dysfunction (BIND) (aka subtle kernicterus) was actually defined by the presence of subtle developmental disabilities without the classical findings of kernicterus [12]. Patients may exhibit neurodevelopmental disabilities with a history of excessive hyperbilirubinemia and prior signs of bilirubin encephalopathy. Subtle kernicterus spectrum disorders may also be associated with conditions related to the findings of classical kernicterus, such as auditory imperception, aphasia, and other neurodevelopmental disorders (e.g., central auditory processing disorders, sensory and sensorimotor integration disorders, hypotonia, ataxia or clumsiness) [12]. An important clinical issue of subtle kernicterus/BIND seems to be auditory neuropathy, defined as impaired auditory brainstem reflexes with normal otoacoustic emissions or cochlear microphonic responses. Auditory brainstem response is said to be absent or abnormal, reflecting damage to the auditory nerve and/or auditory brainstem nuclei [7]. Le Pichon et al. (2017), however, suggested using the term Kernicterus

Spectrum Disorders to encompass all neurological sequelae of bilirubin neurotoxicity, acknowledging that kernicterus is symptomatically broad and diverse [17].

3. Diagnostic Testing

Infants who appear jaundiced should be evaluated with a risk score or total serum/transcutaneous bilirubin measurement [2,18]. The transcutaneous method of measuring bilirubin has the advantage of being less invasive, with results becoming available much more quickly compared to serum measurement and is potentially more cost effective, but this method may not be reliable at bilirubin levels greater than 15 to 20 mg/dL [19]. The bilirubin levels should be interpreted in relation to the infant's age in hours. Recommendations from the American Academy of Pediatrics state that laboratory tests should be ordered for all infants with jaundice who require phototherapy, including neonatal blood type, direct antibody titer/Coombs test, complete blood count, blood smear, and direct/conjugated bilirubin level [2].

In neonates, serum unconjugated bilirubin (UCB) is usually elevated during the first two weeks of postnatal life due to the increased breakdown of fetal erythrocytes, deficient albumin transport to the liver, and decreased conjugation leading to physiological jaundice of the newborn, requiring no treatment [20]. In some newborn infants however, serum levels of unconjugated bilirubin can increase significantly due to impaired postnatal maturation of hepatic transport, impaired conjugation of bilirubin, or augmented hemolysis. This jaundice is pathologic and may lead to death or severe neurodevelopmental complications in survivors [20]. Unconjugated bilirubin levels close to 20 mg/dL have been reported to be related to kernicterus [21].

Measurement of free/unbound bilirubin (i.e., bilirubin not bound to albumin) can also be an important marker of the risk of hyperbilirubinemia. A study by Morioka et al. (2015) involving 18 preterm (<30 weeks) infants (birth weight < 1000 g) diagnosed with kernicterus between 2002 and 2012 based on clinical history, neurological examinations, and laboratory investigations, found the median age at which total bilirubin levels peaked was 28 days after birth. The majority of these infants (16/18) were 14 or more days of age and the latest age recorded for peak total bilirubin levels was 86 days. The median serum total and unbound bilirubin levels in this cohort at that age were 17.0 mg/dL and 1.67×10^{-3} mg/dL, respectively. Nine of 18 infants had high total and unbound bilirubin, while seven of eight infants with low total bilirubin had high unbound bilirubin. The results of this work suggest that chronic high unbound bilirubin levels may help identify early low-birth weight infants at risk of developing kernicterus [22]. Measurement of unbound bilirubin is still not feasible in most parts of the world, but we believe the above-mentioned study emphasizes the importance of developing an accurate method for its determination in clinical practice.

Iskander et al. (2014) performed a longitudinal observational study in which the neurologic status and auditory impairment (automated auditory brainstem response) were evaluated (both at admission and posttreatment) in 193 term/near-term infants that were admitted to hospital for jaundice. Relationships of total serum bilirubin (TSB) and the bilirubin-albumin (B/A) ratio to advancing stages of neurotoxicity were compared using receiver operating characteristic curves. The authors found a stepwise relationship between median and threshold values of TSB and the B/A ratio, and the progression of acute neurotoxicity. However, they concluded that the B/A ratio did not improve the prediction of bilirubin encephalopathy over total serum bilirubin levels alone [23]. Other authors similarly consider a high B/A ratio in preterm infants to be a risk factor and suggest its use in conjunction with TSB for the evaluation and treatment of premature infants with hyperbilirubinemia [24]. Elevated B/A ratios may be especially helpful to predict the risk of bilirubin neurotoxicity in cases of so-called low bilirubin kernicterus in which bilirubin-induced neuronal injury is said to occur at total bilirubin levels that are thought to be non-hazardous with low albumin levels [25]. Novel methods for bilirubin quantification have been developed in recent years. A detailed discussion of these methods is beyond the scope of this article, but the interested reader is referred to the excellent review by Ngashangva et al. (2019) [26].

The above-mentioned methods, although accurate, are fairly expensive, and therefore may not be accessible in low-income countries. The Bilistick method is an in vitro point-of-care diagnostic method for measuring TSB from capillary or venous blood samples [27]. This is a much cheaper method and multiple studies have found it to be an accurate alternative [28,29]. The Bilistick method also has the added advantage of having a much shorter turn-around-time (time interval between specimen collection and reporting of TSB result) compared to serum measurement and even transcutaneous measurement of bilirubin [27].

The bilirubin-induced neurological dysfunction (BIND) score is a nine-point scale assessing mental status, muscle tones, and crying patterns (Table 1). A BIND score of 0 is normal, while BIND scores 1–3, 4–6, and 7–9 are meant to represent mild, moderate, and severe acute bilirubin encephalopathy, respectively [30,31]. El Houchi et al. (2017) studied the ability of the BIND score to predict not only neurologic and auditory disability, but also its relationship to total serum bilirubin concentration. BIND scores of 220 term and near-term infants (117 boys, 103 girls; age range = $0.1 - 13.3$ years) with severe hyperbilirubinemia were obtained at 6- and 8-h intervals. Median highest total serum bilirubin in this cohort was recorded at 29.7 mg/dL, with a range 17–61 mg/dL. The authors found that a BIND score ≥ 4 had a specificity of 87.3% and sensitivity of 97.4% for predicting a poor neurologic outcome, and a specificity and sensitivity of 87.3% and 92.6%, respectively, for predicting long-term hearing impairment. It is worth noting, however, that four infants with total serum bilirubin levels ≥ 36 mg/dL had BIND scores ≤ 3 and normal outcomes at follow-up, while one infant with a low BIND score developed severe auditory neuropathy. Although a positive correlation between BIND scores and total serum bilirubin was observed, the coefficient of determination was not very high ($r^2 = 0.54$, $p < 0.005$). However, they did demonstrate that the risk of severe acute bilirubin encephalopathy increased with increasing total serum bilirubin, especially TSB above 30 mg/dL [30].

Table 1. BIND Score (Cited from Johnson et al. 2009 [31]).

Clinical Parameter	BIND Score
Mental status	
Normal	0
Sleep but arousable, decreased feeding	1
Lethargy, poor suck and/or irritable/jittery with strong suck	2
Semi-coma, unable to feed, seizures, coma	3
Muscle tone	
Normal	0
Persistent mild to moderate hypotonia	1
Hypertonia alternating with hypotonia, beginning arching of neck and trunk on stimulation	2
Persistent retrocollis and opisthotonos—bicycling or twitching of hands and feet	3
Cry pattern	
Normal	0
High pitched when aroused	1
Shrill, difficult to console	2
Inconsolable crying or cry weak or absent	3
TOTAL	Sum of scores from each parameter

4. Neuroimaging

Signal abnormalities are classically reported in the globus pallidus, hippocampus, and cerebellum, but the nature of these signal abnormalities tends to vary with time. MRI studies of infants in the first days to weeks following acute bilirubin encephalopathy onset (i.e., subacute phase) are said to demonstrate an increased T1-signal in the globus pallidus and subthalamic nucleus, while T2-weighted imaging of these regions is often unremarkable or shows subtle T2-hyperintensity [32,33]. In Wang et al.'s (2008) study involving 24 neonates (including two premature infants) who underwent conventional MRI, the main findings were found to be an abnormal bilateral increased signal intensity in the globus pallidus on T1-weighted images without apparent T2-signal changes for 19 of the 24 patients. Of these 19 patients, 10 of them had a high signal intensity on T1-weighted imaging, but normal T2- signal in the subthalamic nucleus [32].

Interestingly, some authors report that the sensitivity and specificity of T1-signal changes to predict kernicterus during the subacute phase is hindered by both the evolving nature of signal abnormalities and confounding signal changes associated with normal myelination [34]. In infants who later show clinical evidence of chronic bilirubin encephalopathy (i.e., kernicterus), the earliest MRI changes tend to show a high T1-signal in the globus pallidus and subthalamic nucleus. It should be noted that an increased T1-signal in these regions can also be seen as part of normal brain development, such as myelination, and patients with kernicterus may also not necessarily show any abnormalities on MRI [35]. Myelinated white matter tracts such as the internal capsule appear relatively hyperintense on T1-weighted images, while grey matter structures such as the globus pallidus tend to be less hyperintense on T1-weighted images because of the longer relaxation time [35]. Therefore, in infants with incomplete myelination, the globus pallidus may appear brighter and may be confused as pathologic increase in T1-signal intensity. Neuroimaging findings therefore need to be interpreted in the context of obtained clinical history, neurological exam findings, and results of serum biomarkers.

The neuroimaging hallmark of kernicterus is said to be the bilateral and symmetric increase of the T2- and/or FLAIR signal in the globus pallidus and subthalamic nucleus. An increased T2 signal may also be seen in the substantia nigra of the midbrain and dentate nucleus of the cerebellum [33].

Data regarding findings from more advanced imaging techniques such as diffusion weighted imaging (DWI) and MR spectroscopy (MRS) are still limited. Wisnowski et al. (2016) reported a case of a 3400 g female neonate born at 41-weeks gestation who presented with jaundice before 24 h of life, followed by lethargy and poor feeding, and a total serum bilirubin of 28 mg/dL. She underwent MRI, where DWI showed restricted diffusion in the superior thalamic radiations, ventroanterior (VA), and ventrolateral (VL) nuclei of the thalamus, hippocampus, substantia nigra, subthalamic nucleus, superior cerebellar peduncle, pontine nuclei, and dentate nucleus of the cerebellum. Interestingly, no apparent diffusion restriction in the globus pallidus or descending corticospinal tracts was appreciated. Apparent diffusion coefficient (ADC) images demonstrated the acute involvement of selected white matter tracts, such as superior cerebellar peduncles and superior thalamic radiations. In addition, ^{1}H-MRS spectra acquired from the right thalamus revealed elevated glutamate/glutamine concentrations [36]. These observations suggest the involvement of cortico-ponto-cerebello-thalamo-cortical pathways. These pathways include descending projections from the motor cortex to the pontine nuclei (i.e., cortico-pontine pathway), and ascending projections from the dentate nucleus to the motor cortex (i.e., the dentato-thalmo-cortical pathway), with the implication that bilirubin toxicity may target not just neurons, but white matter connections as well.

Some studies have suggested that proton (^{1}H)-MRS studies of infants with acute bilirubin encephalopathy and/or severe hyperbilirubinemia can demonstrate decreases in the ratios of N-acetyl-aspartate (NAA) to choline, and NAA to creatine, as well as increases in the ratio of lactate to NAA in the vicinity of the basal ganglia in neonates who go on to develop kernicterus [32,37,38]. Wu et al.'s (2013) study enrolled 11 patients in their neonatal bilirubin encephalopathy group, eight in their neonatal hyperbilirubinemia group, and nine in their age-matched group, all of whom underwent ^{1}H-MRS and conventional MRI studies using a 1.5 tesla whole body MR scanner. The authors observed

NAA/Cr and NAA/Cho peak-area ratios in the basal ganglia to be much lower in the neonatal bilirubin encephalopathy group than in the neonatal hyperbilirubinemia and control groups ($p < 0.05$). Their study did not, however, show any statistically significant differences in the peak-ratios of NAA/Cr and NAA/Cho in the basal ganglia between the neonatal hyperbilirubinemia and control groups ($p > 0.05$) or in the thalamus between the three groups. There was also no statistically significant difference observed in the Cho/Cr ratios in the basal ganglia and thalamus between the three groups [38]. These findings suggest that ^{1}H-MRS can be useful in differentiating infants who go onto develop kernicterus versus those who have severe hyperbilirubinemia but do not go on to develop clinical sequelae. Further research is required to formulate more concrete conclusions regarding the utility of these techniques in the diagnosis of bilirubin encephalopathy and kernicterus.

5. Neuropathology

The most consistent abnormality reported in the literature is atrophy of the globus pallidus, but the hippocampus, thalamus, hypothalamus, and subthalamic nucleus may also display atrophy. Classic full-blown kernicterus typically leads to yellow discoloration of the basal ganglia, especially the globus pallidus, and subthalamic nucleus (see Figure 1). Other susceptible areas include the thalamus, mammillary bodies, CA2 sector of the hippocampus, subiculum, indusium griseum, and uncus. Vulnerable areas in the brainstem include the substantia nigra, oculomotor nucleus, trochlear nucleus, cochlear nucleus, vestibular nucleus, inferior colliculus, and superior olivary complex. Purkinje cells and a dentate nucleus of the cerebellum are also reported to be potentially involved [7,39,40].

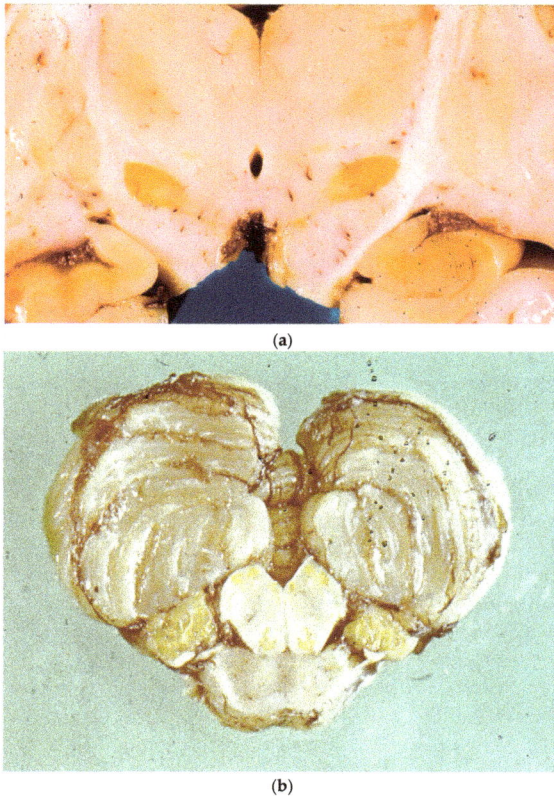

(a)

(b)

Figure 1. *Cont.*

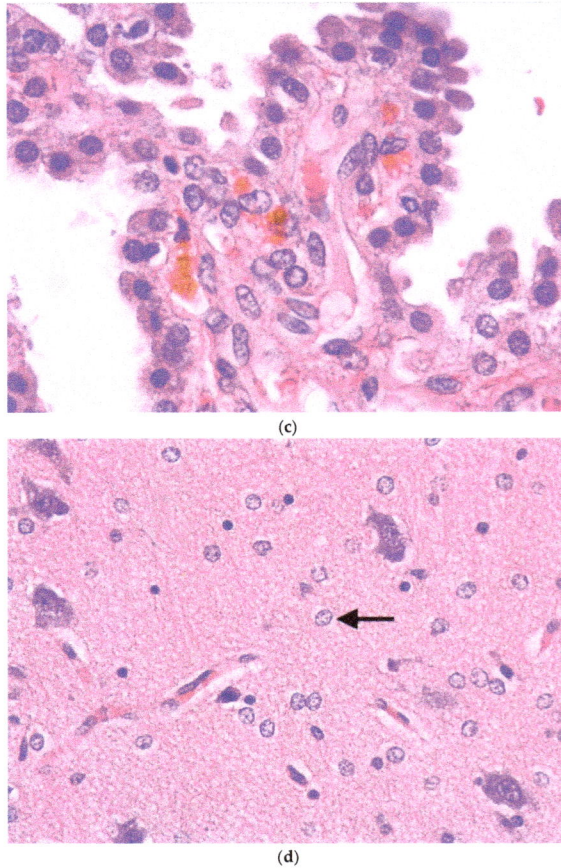

Figure 1. Neuropathologic findings from a patient with kernicterus. (**a**) Yellowish discoloration of subthalamic nucleus and hippocampus; (**b**) discoloration of medullary tegmentum, inferior olives, and cerebellar tonsils; (**c**) cytoplasmic pigment in cells of choroid plexus (20× magnification); (**d**) Alzheimer's type II astrocytes (arrow) in keeping with liver failure (20× magnification).

On microscopic examination, the primary target of injury is neurons. Neuronal changes are those of acute necrosis resembling that seen in hypoxic-ischemic encephalopathy and hypoglycemia. Within a few days after injurious insult, these dead neurons may become encrusted with calcium or iron. Neuronal damage can be found in the lateral and medial nucleus of the globus pallidus, subthalamic nucleus, mammillary bodies, indusium griseum, hippocampus, nucleus of the third and fourth cranial nerves, substantia nigra, and interstitial nucleus of Cajal. Chronic lesions, also referred to as post-kernicteric encephalopathy, display necrosis, vacuolation of the cytoplasm, and prominent neuronal loss, as well as gliosis in the globus pallidus, subthalamic nucleus, and hippocampus [40–42]. With regards to neuronal changes, the earliest (within the first several days of bilirubin-induced injury) neuronal changes consist of swollen granular cytoplasm, often with microvacuolation and the disruption of neuronal and nuclear membranes. Yellow pigment can be prominent within the neuronal cytoplasm. By the end of the first week, dissolution of affected neurons becomes apparent, and nuclear and plasma membranes become poorly defined. In subsequent days to weeks, neuronal loss, often with mineralization, and astrocytosis can be observed. As in other causes of liver injury, Alzheimer's type II astrocytes (Figure 1d) can be found throughout the deep grey matter structures, as well as the neocortex, brainstem, and cerebellum [43–45].

Bilirubin staining is said to be best seen in fresh specimens or in frozen sections, especially in infants who survive several days. The anatomic distribution of this staining includes the globus pallidus, subthalamic nucleus, hippocampus (particularly CA2 and CA3 sectors), substantia nigra, cranial nerve nuclei (particularly oculomotor, facial, vestibular, and cochlear nuclei), superior olivary complex, nuclei of lateral lemniscus, inferior colliculus, reticular formation of pons, inferior olivary nuclei, dentate nucleus of the cerebellum, and anterior horn cells of the spinal cord [43,44,46,47]. This period of prominent brain pigmentation lasts for approximately seven to 10 days, and is accompanied by the commencement of neuronal changes that result in post-kernicteric bilirubin encephalopathy [45,48]. We recently encountered a post-mortem case in our institution (not published) in which pigment was found in cells of choroid plexus (Figure 1c). Brito et al. (2013), in their case report of a 32-week old female with kernicterus, suggested that unconjugated bilirubin increases the vascular density of brain regions associated with kernicterus, such as the hippocampus and corpus striatum, while triggering VEGF and VEGFR-2 immunoreactivity, along with albumin extravasation into the brain parenchyma [48].

White matter abnormalities have also been reported in premature infants with kernicterus. For example, periventricular white matter injury in the form of periventricular leukomalacia has been reported as a frequent occurrence in the context of kernicterus [49]. Our recent postmortem case (not published) of kernicterus also showed evidence of chronic periventricular white matter injury typified by the presence of gliosis, macrophages, and sparse microcalcification in the periventricular white matter. With more diffuse periventricular white matter injury, ventriculomegaly and thinned corpus callosum may be observed [49]. A case report from Brito et al. (2012) of a preterm (32 weeks five days, weight = 1600 g) infant who passed away on the fourth day of life with a diagnosis of kernicterus reported a poorer staining intensity of Luxol-fast blue-periodic acid Schiff in the cerebellar white matter compared to an age-matched non-icteric cerebellum. This poor staining intensity indicated a decreased density of myelinated fibres, in keeping with demyelination. Axonal integrity was further assessed with Bodian-Luxol fast blue stain and revealed axons to be severely affected by hyperbilirubinemia compared to the non-icteric brain [50]. Findings from in vivo and in vitro experiments seem to suggest a decreased number of myelinated axons, decreased thickness of myelin sheaths, and less compact axons with more debris in brains exposed to unconjugated bilirubin [51].

6. Management

Management of patients with kernicterus is directed towards neurodevelopmental sequelae, which entails physical, occupational, speech, and audiological therapies; as well as complications including nutritional difficulties, gastroesophageal reflux, sleep disturbances, hypertonicity, and muscle cramps [12]. Established treatment strategies for acute bilirubin encephalopathy, on the other hand, include phototherapy and exchange transfusion [16]. Traditionally, the decision to start phototherapy has been based on birthweight because of the strong positive correlation that is believed to exist between total serum bilirubin and birthweight [7,52]. Interestingly, a Japanese group revised their treatment criteria for the treatment of preterm hyperbilirubinemic infants. The revisions included classifying newborns based on gestational age at birth or corrected gestational age rather than birthweight as it is gestational age at birth or corrected gestational age that is associated with organ maturation. Additionally, the treatment options created were standard phototherapy, intensive phototherapy, and albumin therapy and/or exchange transfusion. Finally, the decision to initiate any of these therapies is based on the total serum bilirubin and unbound bilirubin reference values for gestational age (in weeks) at birth for < 7 days after birth and ≥ 7 days of age [53]. Measurement of unbound bilirubin is still not easily achievable in other parts of the world. We believe that further studies are necessary to accurately determine the efficacy of administering these therapies based on bilirubin levels, as well as the bilirubin/albumin ratio. It has also been argued that the efficacy of treatments for acute bilirubin encephalopathy has generated overconfidence in the medical environment about the management of severe hyperbilirubinemia [54]. This can lead to an increased risk of neurological sequelae, even in western countries. Prevention of tragedies that can arise from severe hyperbilirubinemia and kernicterus requires the implementation of evidence-based guidelines for the management of neonatal jaundice [54]. What is also needed are more devices like the Bili-stick that are relatively cheap, easy to use, and accurate for distinguishing between healthy children and those at risk, especially for low-income countries where the prevalence of kernicterus is higher.

7. Conclusions

Herein, the authors have described the range of clinical, radiological, and neuropathological changes features (summarized in Box 1) that can be encountered in patients with bilirubin encephalopathy/kernicterus. Further research is required to accurately determine the efficacy of available treatment options on various parameters, including total serum bilirubin levels and bilirubin-albumin ratio, as well as whether other more innovative therapeutic options are possible.

Box 1. Key Concepts—Acute Bilirubin Encephalopathy (ABE) and Kernicterus.

Risk Factors:
Low gestational age, low birth weight, hemolysis, sepsis, cephalohematoma, easy bruising, exclusive breast feeding.

Clinical Presentation:
ABE: feeding, lethargy, hypotonia and/or hypertonia, high-pitched cry, retrocollis and opisthotonus, setting sun sign, fever, seizures, death.
Kernicterus: abnormal motor control, abnormal movements, abnormal muscle tone, oculomotor impairments, enamel dysplasia, auditory complications.

Neuroimaging highlights:
ABE: Increased T1-signal intensity in globus pallidus and subthalamic nucleus.
Kernicterus: Increased T2/FLAIR signal intensity in globus pallidus and subthalamic nucleus; possible increased T2-signal in substantia nigra and cerebellar dentate nucleus.

Neuropathological Findings:
- Atrophy of the globus pallidus, hippocampus, thalamus, hypothalamus, and subthalamic nucleus.
- Yellow discoloration of the basal ganglia, especially the globus pallidus and subthalamic nucleus.
- Neuronal necrosis followed by dissolution.

Management:
ABE: Phototherapy, exchange transfusion.
Kernicterus: Supportive management of neurological sequelae.

Author Contributions: Preparation of manuscript: S.D.; Preparation of figures: F.K.H.v.L.

Funding: This review received no external funding.

Conflicts of Interest: The authors declare no conflict of interest.

References

1. Olusanya, B.O.; Ogunlesi, T.A.; Slusher, T.M. Why is kernicterus still a major cause of death and disability in low-income and middle-income countries? *Arch. Dis. Child.* **2014**, *99*, 1117–1121. [CrossRef] [PubMed]
2. Muchowski, K.E. Evaluation and treatment of neonatal hyperbilirubinemia. *Am. Fam. Physician* **2014**, *89*, 873–878. [PubMed]
3. Bhardwaj, K.; Locke, T.; Biringer, A.; Booth, A.; Darling, E.K.; Dougan, S.; Harrison, J.; Hill, S.; Johnson, A.; Makin, S.; et al. Newborn Bilirubin Screening for Preventing Severe Hyperbilirubinemia and Bilirubin Encephalopathy: A Rapid Review. *Curr. Pediatr. Rev.* **2017**, *13*, 67–90. [CrossRef] [PubMed]
4. Chang, P.W.; Newman, T.B.; Maisels, M.J. Update on Predicting Severe Hyperbilirubinemia and Bilirubin Neurotoxicity Risks in Neonates. *Curr. Pediatr. Rev.* **2017**, *13*, 181–187. [CrossRef] [PubMed]

5. Olusanya, B.O.; Kaplan, M.; Hansen, W.R. Neonatal hyperbilirubinemia: A global perspective. *Lancet Child Adolesc. Health* **2018**, *2*, 610–620. [CrossRef]
6. Shapiro, S.M. Bilirubin toxicity in the developing nervous system. *Pediatr. Neurol.* **2003**, *29*, 410–421. [CrossRef] [PubMed]
7. Shapiro, S.M. Definition of the Clinical Spectrum of Kernicterus and Bilirubin-Induced Neurologic Dysfunction (BIND). *J. Perinatol.* **2005**, *25*, 54–59. [CrossRef] [PubMed]
8. Slusher, T.M.; Owa, J.A.; Painter, M.J.; Shapiro, S.M. The Kernicteric Facies: Facial Features of Acute Bilirubin Encephalopathy. *Pediatr. Neurol.* **2001**, *44*, 153–154. [CrossRef] [PubMed]
9. Amin, S.B.; Bhutani, V.K.; Watchko, J.F. Apnea in acute bilirubin encephalopathy. *Semin. Perinatal.* **2014**, *38*, 407–411. [CrossRef] [PubMed]
10. Amin, S.B.; Charafeddine, L.; Guillet, R. Transient bilirubin encephalopathy and apnea of prematurity in 28 to 32 weeks gestational age infants. *J. Perinatol.* **2005**, *25*, 386–390. [CrossRef] [PubMed]
11. Gkoltsiou, K.; Tzoufi, M.; Counsell, S.; Rutherford, M.; Cowan, F. Serial brain MRI and ultrasound findings: Relation to gestational age, bilirubin level, neonatal neurologic status and neurodevelopmental outcome in infants at risk of kernicterus. *Early Hum. Dev.* **2008**, *84*, 829–838. [CrossRef] [PubMed]
12. Shaprio, S.M. Chronic bilirubin encephalopathy: Diagnosis and outcome. *Semin. Fetal Neonatal Med.* **2010**, *15*, 157–163. [CrossRef] [PubMed]
13. Uziel, A.; Marot, M.; Pujol, R. The Gunn rat: An experimental model for central deafness. *Acta Otolaryngol.* **1983**, *95*, 651–656. [CrossRef] [PubMed]
14. Olds, C.; Oghalai, J.S. Bilirubin-Induced Audiologic Injury in Preterm Infants. *Clin. Perinatol.* **2016**, *43*, 313–323. [CrossRef] [PubMed]
15. Matkin, N.; Carhart, R. Auditory profiles associated with Rh incompatibility. *Arch. Otolaryngol.* **1966**, *84*, 502–513. [CrossRef] [PubMed]
16. Rose, J.; Vassar, R. Movement disorders due to bilirubin toxicity. *Semin. Fetal Neonatal Med.* **2015**, *20*, 20–25. [CrossRef] [PubMed]
17. Le Pichon, J.B.; Riordan, S.M.; Watchko, J.; Shapiro, S.M. The Neurological Sequelae of Neonatal Hyperbilirubinemia: Definitions, Diagnosis and Treatment of the Kernicterus Spectrum Disorders (KSDs). *Curr. Pediatr. Rev.* **2017**, *13*, 199–209. [PubMed]
18. American Academy of Pediatrics. Management of hyperbilirubinemia in the newborn infant 35 or more weeks of gestation. *Pediatrics* **2004**, *114*, 297–316. [CrossRef]
19. Taylor, J.A.; Burgos, A.E.; Flaherman, V.; Chung, E.K.; Simpson, E.A.; Goyal, N.K.; Von Kohorn, I.; Dhepyasuwan, N. Discrepancies between transcutaneous and serum bilirubin measurements. *Pediatrics* **2015**, *135*, 224–231. [CrossRef] [PubMed]
20. Brito, M.A.; Silva, R.F.M.; Brites, D. Cell response to hyperbilirubinemia: A journey along key molecular events. In *New Trends in Brain Research*; Chen, F.J., Ed.; Nova Science Publishers, Inc.: New York, NY, USA, 2006; pp. 1–38.
21. Odutolu, Y.; Emmerson, A.J. Low bilirubin kernicterus with sepsis and hypoalbuminemia. *BMJ Case Rep.* **2013**. [CrossRef] [PubMed]
22. Morioka, I.; Nakamura, H.; Koda, T.; Sakai, H.; Kurokawa, D.; Yonetani, M.; Morisawa, T.; Katayama, Y.; Wada, H.; Funato, M.; et al. Serum unbound bilirubin as a predictor for clinical kernicterus in extremely low birth weight infants at a late age in the neonatal intensive care unit. *Brain Dev.* **2015**, *37*, 753–757. [CrossRef] [PubMed]
23. Iskander, I.; Gamaleldin, R.; El Houchi, S.; El Shenawy, A.; Seoud, I.; El Gharbawi, N.; Abou-Youssef, H.; Aravkin, A.; Wennberg, R.P. Serum bilirubin and bilirubin/albumin ratio as predictors of bilirubin encephalopathy. *Pediatrics* **2014**, *134*, e1330–e1339. [CrossRef] [PubMed]
24. Hulzebos, C.V.; van Imhoff, D.E.; Bos, A.F.; Ahlfors, C.E.; Verkade, H.J.; Dijk, P.H. Usefulness of bilirubin/albumin ratio for predicting bilirubin-induced neurotoxicity in preterm infants. *Arch. Dis. Child.-Fetal Neonatal Ed.* **2008**, *93*, F384–F388. [CrossRef] [PubMed]
25. Watchko, J.F. Bilirubin Induced Neurotoxicity in the Preterm Neonate. *Clin. Perinatol.* **2016**, *43*, 297–311. [CrossRef] [PubMed]
26. Ngashangva, L.; Bacha, V.; Goswami, P. Development of new methods for determination of bilirubin. *J. Pharm. Biomed. Anal.* **2019**, *5*, 272–285. [CrossRef] [PubMed]

27. Boo, N.Y.; Chang, Y.F.; Leong, Y.X.; Tok, Z.Y.; Hooi, L.C.; Chee, S.C.; Latif, Z.A. The point-of-care Bilistick method has very short turn-around-time and high accuracy at lower cutoff levels to predict laboratory-measured TSB. *Pediatr. Res.* **2019**. [CrossRef] [PubMed]

28. Greco, C.; Iskander, I.F.; Akmal, D.M.; El Houchi, S.Z.; Khairy, D.A.; Bedogni, G.; Wennberg, R.P.; Tiribelli, C.; Coda Zabetta, C.D. Comparison between Bilistick System and transcutaneous bilirubin in assessing total bilirubin serum concentration in jaundiced newborns. *J. Perinatol.* **2017**, *37*, 1028–1031. [CrossRef] [PubMed]

29. Rohsiswatmo, R.; Oswari, H.; Amandito, R.; Sjakti, H.A.; Windiastuti, E.; Roeslani, R.D.; Barchia, I. Agreement test of transcutaneous bilirubin and bilistick with serum bilirubin in preterm infants receiving phototherapy. *BMC Pediatr.* **2018**, *18*, 315. [CrossRef] [PubMed]

30. El Houchi, S.Z.; Iskander, I.; Gamaleldin, R.; El Shenawy, A.; Seoud, I.; Abou-Youssef, H.; Wennberg, R.P. Prediction of 3- to 5-Month Outcomes from Signs of Acute Bilirubin Toxicity in Newborn Infants. *J. Pediatr.* **2017**, *183*, 51–55. [CrossRef] [PubMed]

31. Johnson, L.; Bhutani, V.K.; Karp, K.; Sivieri, E.M.; Shapiro, S.M. Clinical report from the pilot USA Kernicterus Registry (1992 to 2004). *J. Perinatol.* **2009**, *29*, S25–S45. [CrossRef] [PubMed]

32. Wang, X.; Wu, W.; Hou, B.L.; Zhang, P.; Chineah, A.; Liu, F.; Liao, W. Studying neonatal bilirubin encephalopathy with conventional MRI, MRS, and DWI. *Neuroradiology* **2008**, *50*, 885–893. [CrossRef] [PubMed]

33. Wiskownski, J.L.; Panigraphy, A.; Painter, M.J.; Watchko, J.F. Magnetic resonance imaging of bilirubin encephalopathy: Current limitations and future promise. *Semin. Perinatol.* **2014**, *38*, 422–428. [CrossRef] [PubMed]

34. Shapiro, S.M. Kernicterus. In *Care of the Jaundiced Neonate*; Stevenson, D.K., Maisels, M.J., Watchko, J.F., Eds.; McGraw-Hill: New York, NY, USA, 2012; pp. 229–242.

35. Barkovich, A.J. MR of the normal neonatal brain: Assessment of deep structures. *AJNR Am. J. Neuroradiol.* **1998**, *19*, 1397–1403. [PubMed]

36. Wisnowski, J.L.; Panigrahy, A.; Painter, M.J.; Watchko, J.F. Magnetic Resonance Imaging Abnormalities in Advanced Acute Bilirubin Encephalopathy Highlight Dentato-Thalamo-Cortical Pathways. *J. Pediatr.* **2016**, *174*, 260–263. [CrossRef] [PubMed]

37. Groenendaal, F.; van der Grond, J.; de Vries, L.S. Cerebral metabolism in severe neonatal hyperbilirubinemia. *Pediatrics* **2004**, *114*, 291–294. [CrossRef] [PubMed]

38. Wu, W.; Zhang, P.; Wang, X.; Chineah, A.; Lou, M. Usefulness of ^{1}H-MRS in differentiating bilirubin encephalopathy from severe hyperbilirubinemia in neonates. *J. Magn. Reson. Imaging* **2013**, *38*, 634–640. [CrossRef] [PubMed]

39. López-Corella, E.; Ibarra-González, I.; Fernández-Lainez, C.; Rodríguez-Weber, M.Á.; Guillén-Lopez, S.; Belmont-Martínez, L.; Agüero-Linares, D.; Vela-Amieva, M. Kernicterus in a boy with ornithine transcarbamylase deficiency: A case report. *Neuropathology* **2017**, *37*, 586–590. [CrossRef] [PubMed]

40. Adle-Biassette, H.; Harding, B.; Golden, J.A. *Developmental Neuropathology*; John Wiley and Sons Ltd.: Oxford, UK, 2018.

41. Friede, R.L. Kernicterus (Bilirubin encephalopathy). In *Developmental Neuropathology*; Springer: Berlin, Germany, 1989; pp. 113–124.

42. Kinney, H.C.; Armstrong, D.D. Perinatal neuropathology. In *Greenfield's Neuropathology*; Graham, D.I., Lantos, P.L., Eds.; Arnold: London, UK, 2002; pp. 519–606.

43. Ahdab-Barmada, M.; Moossy, J. The neuropathology of kernicterus in the premature neonate: Diagnostic problems. *J. Neuropathol. Exp. Neurol.* **1984**, *43*, 45–56. [CrossRef] [PubMed]

44. Turkel, S.B. Autopsy findings associated with neonatal hyperbilirubinemia. *Clin. Perinatol.* **1990**, *17*, 381–396. [CrossRef]

45. Perlman, J.M.; Rogers, B.B.; Burns, D. Kernicteric findings at autopsy in two sick near term infants. *Pediatrics* **1997**, *99*, 612–615. [CrossRef] [PubMed]

46. Connolly, A.M.; Volpe, J.J. Clinical features of bilirubin encephalopathy. *Clin. Perinatol.* **1990**, *17*, 371–379. [CrossRef]

47. Hayashi, M.; Satoh, J.; Sakamoto, K.; Morimatsu, Y. Clinical and neuropathological findings in severe athetoid cerebral palsy: A comparative study of globo-Luysian and thalamo-putaminal groups. *Brain Dev.* **1991**, *13*, 47–51. [CrossRef]

48. Brito, M.A.; Pereira, P.; Barroso, C.; Aronica, E.; Brites, D. New autopsy findings in different brain regions of a preterm neonate with kernicterus: Neurovascular alterations and up-regulation of efflux transporters. *Pediatr. Neurol.* **2013**, *49*, 431–438. [CrossRef] [PubMed]

49. Watcko, J.F.; Maisels, M.J. The enigma of low bilirubin kernicterus in premature infants: Why does it still occur and is it preventable? *Semin. Perinatol.* **2014**, *38*, 397–406. [CrossRef] [PubMed]

50. Brito, M.A.; Zurolo, E.; Pereira, P.; Barroso, C.; Aronica, E.; Brites, D. Cerebellar axon/myelin loss, axonal sprouting, and neuronal increased in vascular endothelial growth factor in a preterm infant with kernicterus. *J. Child Neurol.* **2012**, *27*, 615–624. [CrossRef] [PubMed]

51. Lakovic, K.; Ai, J.; D'Abbondanza, J.; Tariq, A.; Sabri, M.; Alarfaj, A.K.; Vasdev, P.; Macdonald, R.L. Bilirubin and its oxidation products damage brain white matter. *J. Cereb. Blood Flow Metab.* **2014**, *34*, 1837–1847. [CrossRef] [PubMed]

52. van der Schoor, L.W.; Dijk, P.H.; Verkade, H.J.; Kamsma, A.C.; Schreuder, A.B.; Groen, H.; Hulzebos, C.V. Unconjugated free bilirubin in preterm infants. *Early Hum. Dev.* **2017**, *106–107*, 25–32. [CrossRef] [PubMed]

53. Morioka, I. Hyperbilubinemia in preterm infants in Japan: New treatment criteria. *Pediatr. Int.* **2018**, *60*, 684–690. [CrossRef] [PubMed]

54. Bhuntani, V.K.; Johnson, L. Synopsis report from the pilot USA Kernicterus Registry. *J. Perinatol.* **2009**, *29*, S4–S7. [CrossRef] [PubMed]

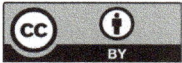

diagnostics

MDPI

Review

Sialidosis: A Review of Morphology and Molecular Biology of a Rare Pediatric Disorder

Aiza Khan [1] and Consolato Sergi [1,2,*]

[1] Department of Laboratory Medicine and Pathology (5B4.09), University of Alberta, 8440 112 St NW, Edmonton, AB T6G 2B7, Canada; draizakhan@gmail.com

[2] Department of Pediatrics, Stollery Children's Hospital, University of Alberta Hospital, Edmonton, AB T6G 2B7, Canada

* Correspondence: sergi@ualberta.ca; Tel.: +1-780-407-7951; Fax: +1-780-407-3009

Received: 23 February 2018; Accepted: 22 April 2018; Published: 25 April 2018

Abstract: Sialidosis (MIM 256550) is a rare, autosomal recessive inherited disorder, caused by α-*N*-acetyl neuraminidase deficiency resulting from a mutation in the neuraminidase gene (*NEU1*), located on 6p21.33. This genetic alteration leads to abnormal intracellular accumulation as well as urinary excretion of sialyloligosaccharides. A definitive diagnosis is made after the identification of a mutation in the *NEU1* gene. So far, 40 mutations of *NEU1* have been reported. An association exists between the impact of the individual mutations and the severity of clinical presentation of sialidosis. According to the clinical symptoms, sialidosis has been divided into two subtypes with different ages of onset and severity, including sialidosis type I (normomorphic or mild form) and sialidosis type II (dysmorphic or severe form). Sialidosis II is further subdivided into (i) congenital; (ii) infantile; and (iii) juvenile. Despite being uncommon, sialidosis has enormous clinical relevance due to its debilitating character. A complete understanding of the underlying pathology remains a challenge, which in turn limits the development of effective therapeutic strategies. Furthermore, in the last few years, some atypical cases of sialidosis have been reported as well. We herein attempt to combine and discuss the underlying molecular biology, the clinical features, and the morphological patterns of sialidosis type I and II.

Keywords: sialidosis; neuraminidase; sialidosis I; sialidosis II; lysosomal storage disease; lysosomal exocytosis

1. Introduction

Sialidosis, an autosomal recessive disorder, occurs due to a structural defect in the neuraminidase gene and is characterized by abnormal tissue accumulation as well as urinary excretion of sialylated oligosaccharides and glycolipids [1].

The human neuraminidase gene is located at chromosome band 6p21.3, where the *HLA* locus is also reported to be located [2]. Until 1977, deficiency of Neuraminidase 1 (NEU1) was thought to be associated with classical mucolipidosis I, a severe and rapidly progressive lysosomal storage disease with onset at birth or shortly after birth [3,4]. In 1977, the term sialidosis was first used to describe the syndrome of two siblings having a visual impairment and mild neurological manifestations that slowly developed in their adolescence. Enzymatic assays in cultured fibroblasts and leukocytes from these siblings exhibited an isolated deficiency of NEU1 [3,4]. Later, Sialidosis was classified into two types: Sialidosis Type I (normomorphic) and Sialidosis Type II (dysmorphic) [5]. In this study, we review the underlying genetics and molecular mechanisms of sialidosis and their correlation with clinical and morphological findings.

2. Background

Sialidase (neuraminidase, EC 3.2.1.18) catalyzes the hydrolysis of terminal sialic acid residues of glycoconjugates. Sialidase has been extensively studied in viruses and bacteria. In these microorganisms, its function is to destroy the sialic acid-containing receptors at the surface of host cells to mobilize bacterial nutrients. In mammals, three types of sialidases have been reported, including the lysosomal, plasma membrane, and cytosolic localized enzymes [1].

In human lysosomes, the degradation of complex macromolecular substrates requires the synergistic action of multiple hydrolases that act synergistically to carry out the degradation process of complex macromolecular substrates efficiently. One such efficient catalytic team is formed by three hydrolases which are ubiquitous, but differentially expressed: the serine carboxypeptidase, protective protein/cathepsin A (PPCA), the sialidase, Neuraminidase-1 (NEU1), and the glycosidase β-Galactosidase (β-GAL) [6]. The different expression of three enzymes can be explained by the fact that deficiency of each leads to three distinct lysosomal storage disorders (LSDs): galactosialidosis (GS) or PPCA deficiency with a secondary combined deficiency of NEU1 and β-GAL, sialidosis or NEU1 deficiency, and GM1-gangliosidosis (GM1) or β-GAL deficiency. Each disease is inherited as an autosomal recessive trait and is distinguished by variable clinical phenotypes, ranging from congenital forms to infantile/juvenile forms. All three present as a systemic disease, involving visceral organs, bone, cartilage, muscle and the nervous system [6].

Catalytic activation of NEU1 is PPCA dependent: The function of NEU1 is to initiate the catabolism glycoproteins and glycolipids, by cleaving their terminal sialic acids. For this, NEU1 depends on its interaction with the auxiliary protein protective protein/cathepsin A (PPCA). PPCA is essential for the stability of NEU1 and acts as a molecular chaperone for the subcellular localization and compartmentalization [7]. It can be assumed that NEU1 mutations that affect its interaction with PPCA may also lead to disease, even if the residues forming the active site of the enzyme remain intact [8]. In fact, researchers using the crystal structures of bacterial sialidases as templates have investigated numerous NEU1 amino acid substitutions related to different clinical phenotypes. Most of those substitutions appear to be located at the core surface of the molecule, demonstrating that they may affect the interaction of NEU1 with its chaperone PPCA. Three pathogenic mutations, F260Y, L270F, and A298V, gathered at the surface of the bacterial sialidases. These enzymes were correctly synthesized yet degraded instantly since the resulting proteins failed to associate with PPCA [9]. A putative region of interaction between NEU1 and PPCA was noticed after a careful study of the hydrodynamic properties of these two proteins. This region appeared to be crucial for NEU1 binding to the precursor form of PPCA. Therefore, *NEU1* mutations affecting amino acids within this domain may affect the stability of the enzyme and subsequent PPCA-mediated transportation to lysosomes [7–9]. It is crucial to remember that a primary defect of PPCA results in the lysosomal disorder galactosialidosis [2]. The similarity in the clinical symptoms of these two disorders can be attributed to the fact that the absence of functional PPCA results in a near-complete secondary deficiency of NEU1 [10].

Mechanisms of Pathogenesis in Sialidosis explained with the help of the Mouse Model: The *Neu1−/−* knockout (KO) mouse model is helpful in understanding the underlying molecular mechanism(s) of sialidosis. *Neu1−/−* mice demonstrated NEU1 as a negative regulator of lysosomal exocytosis. It was observed that in hematopoietic cells, NEU1 negatively regulates lysosomal exocytosis by processing the sialic acids on the lysosomal membrane protein 1 (LAMP1). LAMP1 is an integral membrane protein and plays a useful role in the docking of lysosomes at the plasma membrane (PM). Deficiency or impaired NEU1 activity causes defective processing of the sialic acids on LAMP1, causing accumulation of LAMP1 in an over-sialylated state with a prolonged half-life. This accumulation of over-sialylated LAMP1 increases the number of LAMP1-marked lysosomes that dock at the PM, poised to engage in lysosomal exocytosis upon an influx of calcium. LAMP1's essential function in the docking of lysosomes to the PM has been further supported by the fact that silencing *LAMP1* in NEU1-deficient cells normalize the number of lysosomes docked at the PM and thus decreased the extent of lysosomal exocytosis. Hence, NEU1 loss of function ultimately results in the excessive extracellular release of lysosomal luminal contents from deficient cells of several tissues and organs (Figure 1). Excessive lysosomal exocytosis has now been associated with various pathological manifestations which are characteristic of sialidosis, including its role in neurodegeneration and links with Alzheimer's disease, hearing loss, muscle atrophy and splenomegaly [11]. Moreover, phagocytosis in macrophages, which is regulated by NEU1, as well as NEU1-dependent regulation of insulin signaling are the other pathways that have been considered as additional pathological mechanisms involved in the NEU1 loss of function of the organs [12].

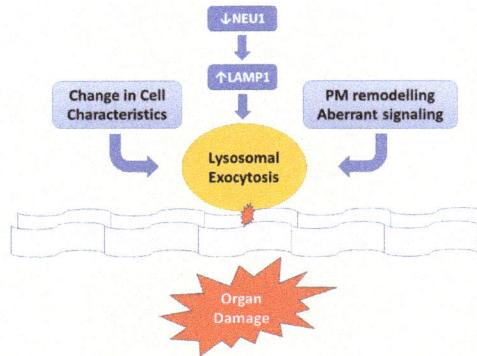

Figure 1. Schematic representation demonstrating downstream of NEU1 deficiency leads to LAMP1 accumulation causing an increased number of lysosomes at the plasmatic membrane (PM) resulting in exacerbated lysosomal exocytosis. Lysosomal-associated membrane protein 1 (LAMP1), aka lysosome-associated membrane glycoprotein 1 or CD107a, is a protein that in humans is determined by the *LAMP1* gene. This abnormal release of lysosomal content causes extracellular PM remodeling. Hence changes in cell characteristics take place with subsequent organ pathogenesis.

3. Morphological and Clinical Aspects of Sialidosis and *NEU1* Mutation(s)

3.1. Method of Study Selection, Criteria, and Data Extraction

Initially, an electronic search was done on Google Scholar, Scopus, and PUBMED. The search was conducted between the time of January 1980 to January 2018. The words used were sialidosis I, sialidosis II, congenital sialidosis, infantile sialidosis, juvenile sialidosis and combinations of these words. In the next step, reference lists of the publications were checked to identify any additional studies. The search was limited to studies published in English in the open literature in peer-reviewed journals.

Cases of sialidosis I typically present later in life (second to third decade); therefore, sialidosis I was discussed briefly in this study. However, for sialidosis II, all cases found were included in the paper since this condition is present in the pediatric group of patients.

Sialidosis (MIM #256550) is known as an autosomal recessive inherited disease. However numerous times, genetic alterations have been found in *NEU1* of unrelated sialidosis patients. So far, more than 40 mutations within the *NEU1* gene have been identified in patients with sialidosis types I and II. Age of onset and severity of the clinical manifestations are paralleled with *NEU1* mutations and the level of residual neuraminidase activity, demonstrating the existence of significant genotype-phenotype correlation in sialidosis.

NEU1 protein variants have been categorized into three groups based on biochemical properties. In the first group, the mutant enzyme stays catalytically inactive and does not localize to the lysosomes; whereas in the second group, the mutant protein localizes to the lysosomes yet is enzymatically inactive.

Finally, in the third group, the mutant protein has residual activity and localizes to the lysosomes. An association appears to exist between individual mutations and the clinical severity of sialidosis [7]. In the least severe form of sialidosis, the modification is thought to cause a decrease in sialidase activity. However, mutant sialidase has residual activity as well as localizing to the lysosomes. Hence, leading to sialidosis I.

3.2. Sialidosis I

Also known as cherry-red spot myoclonus syndrome, type I sialidosis is the less severe, non-neuropathic subtype of this disease. Patients typically exhibit symptoms in the second or third decade of life. Symptoms may include gait abnormalities, decreased visual acuity, or both. Patients usually have no physical defects. Their intelligence level may range from normal to slightly impaired [13]. Myoclonus is an essential feature of sialidosis I, which over the course of the disease tends to get disabling. Precipitating factors may include light touch, sound stimuli, voluntary movements, passive joint movements, voluntary movements, and dysarthria. Action myoclonus, intentional tremors, cerebellar ataxia, and hyperreflexia are the other commonly found symptoms [14]. Muscle strength may remain normal. However, hypotonia can be seen. In some cases, the patients may become wheelchair-bound as the disease progresses [7]. Laboratory tests for sialidosis include a thin-layer chromatography test that is a useful screening test to find an abnormal urinary oligosaccharide pattern. Peripheral blood smear or bone marrow smear may show the presence of storage granules in lymphocytes. Deficiency of the lysosomal sialidase activity (neuraminidase) can be demonstrated in cultured skin fibroblasts obtained from a skin biopsy and is an important diagnostic step. Importantly, in enzymatic studies, sialidosis is differentiated from galactosialidosis by analyzing the enzymatic activity of β-galactosidase which should be normal. The final diagnosis is made after whole genome sequencing. As mentioned earlier, symptoms and their extent of severity are closely associated with the type of *NEU1* mutations involved and subsequently the levels of residual enzyme activity [15].

Pathologically, cytoplasmic accumulation of sialyloligosaccharides has been observed in many neurons in the central nervous systems (CNS) of sialidosis patients. Moreover, neuroradiological imaging studies frequently reveal diffuse brain atrophy in the advanced stage of sialidosis type I, particularly of the cerebellar area [16]. However, initial neuroradiological investigations can be unremarkable in sialidosis 1. Studies also suggest that the major clinical effects seen are caused by changes at a level above the brainstem [17–20]. Further investigation in this area will help in understanding the underlying pathological mechanism which will consequently lead to the availability of better therapeutic approaches.

Atypical Cases of Sialidosis I

In the last decade, one crucial observation regarding sialidosis I is the presence of isolated instances of action myoclonus. Myoclonus, which is considered an essential feature of sialidosis I, has been seen in patients in the absence of other classic symptoms (macular cherry-red spot and sialyloligosacchariduria). After whole genome sequencing, mutations in *NEU1* were identified. This aspect elucidates the fact that mutations affecting NEU1 activity can exist in the absence of other clinical signs that are characteristic of sialidosis [21]. This aspect warrants further studies in this area to investigate if there are more cases of sialidosis I than initially predicted.

3.3. Sialidosis II

Based on the age at onset of the symptoms, type II sialidosis is further divided into three subtypes: (i) congenital or hydropic (in utero); (ii) infantile (0–12 months); and (iii) juvenile (2–20 years) [7,22].

The congenital or hydropic subtype: Profoundly severe mutational alterations may lead to a complete absence of lysosomal neuraminidase and are lethal during fetal development or at birth. The congenital type of sialidosis, which is the severe form of the disease, is thought to be the result of such mutations. It manifests itself prenatally and is characterized by ascites and hydrops fetalis, hepatomegaly and stillbirths or death at a very early age [7]. Table 1 summarizes the cases of congenital sialidosis reported from 1979 until now (cases presented before 1979 can be found in a previous review [5]). It can be observed that hydrops, ascites, and edema are the distinguishing features of the severe, congenital group of the disease, followed by coarse features, dysostosis multiplex, and hepatosplenomegaly. Renal involvement, cardiac anomalies, ophthalmic finding, myoclonus, inguinal hernia, telangiectasias, petechiae, bluish to purpuric macules and hydrocephalus are the clinical features that may infrequently manifest [9,22–46]. Studies reporting histopathological features of congenital sialidosis are limited. In one study, light microscopy of fetal tissues (after pregnancy was terminated at 20 weeks) exhibited vacuolation in the liver, bone marrow, kidney, and brain. In addition, an abnormal pattern of vacuolations was also present in the endocrine organs such as the thyroid gland, adrenal gland, hypophysis, testes as well as in the thymus. Moreover, vacuolation of the placenta demonstrated that in congenital sialidosis abnormal storage takes place during the early fetal period [36]. Figure 2 illustrates vacuolation of placenta, spleen, and thymus of a patient with congenital sialidosis.

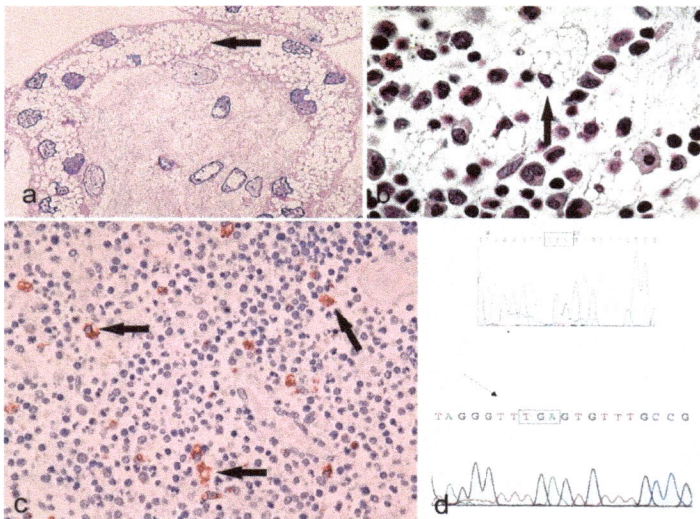

Figure 2. Microphotographs **a–c** showing the vacuolar degeneration of syncytium-trophoblast of a placenta (Hematoxylin & Eosin staining, 400×), bone marrow (Hematoxylin & Eosin staining, 630×, the arrow points to a cell with margination of the nucleus due to an engulfment of the cytoplasm with undigested material), and thymus (Anti-CD68 immunostaining, 200× with the arrows highlighting the macrophages) from a sialidosis pregnancy. The chromatogram in **d** shows the genetic alteration of the sialidosis gene.

Infantile/juvenile subtype: It has been suggested that *NEU1* mutations in which mutant enzymes localize to the lysosomes yet stay enzymatically inactive lead to the infantile/juvenile subtype of sialidosis II, which is characterized by the development of progressive mucopolysaccharidosis-like phenotype; Patients presenting with coarse facies, visceromegaly, dysostosis multiplex, vertebral deformities, mental retardation [7,47–55]. Table 2 summarizes the clinical features of the infantile/juvenile subtype. Skeletal abnormalities, mainly dysostosis multiplex appear to be a consistent feature of infantile/juvenile phenotypes, along with coarse facies, hepatosplenomegaly, and severe mental retardation. Ocular manifestations, including cherry red spots, cataracts, nystagmus, strabismus, and corneal clouding are common as well while hypotonia, renal involvement, and cardiac anomalies are relatively infrequent findings. It is noticeable that earlier onset of disease has a fulminant course. While in late-onset, the patient may survive for more extended periods (only four patients survived for more than two decades). Hearing loss and ataxia may present in the late onset of infantile/juvenile form and tend to worsen with time. One case of sialidosis II was reported in the last decade, in which the patient developed myoclonic seizures at the age of 17, followed by dysphagia and dysphonia. There was a marked delay in motor and cognitive functions since childhood which worsened over time. However, the patient was able to achieve an elementary school education. At the time of diagnosis, the patient was 30 years old and bedridden, with an advanced degree of mental deficiency. It is notable that the patient was able to achieve education demonstrates that her cognitive delay was not as severe in childhood but progressed with age [55]. This detail seems essential and may aid in future developing therapeutic interventions in this area. Also, it is noteworthy that myoclonus, which is considered a characteristic of sialidosis I, is found in both Congenital as well as Infantile/Juvenile subtypes. (Tables 1 and 2).

NEU1 knockout model *Neu1*−/− mice developed a systemic and neurodegenerative condition that is comparable to the early onset of sialidosis II [10] thus helping in understanding the clinical manifestation of this disease. Some typical clinical features that have been studied and explained are as follows. Hepatosplenomegaly is a fairly standard feature in sialidosis II. Enlargement of the spleen observed in *Neu1*−/−mice is consistent with this finding. Histological studies of spleens in mutant mice showed a time-dependent expansion of total splenic cell counts along with an increased number of erythroid precursors and megakaryocytes. Along with these changes in the spleen, an increased number of hematopoietic progenitors in the peripheral blood and an overall lower number of these cells in the bone marrow (BM) was found. Thus, indicating extramedullary hematopoiesis (EMH) as the possible cause of splenic hypertrophy in *Neu1*−/−. Furthermore, immunohistochemical studies of mutant livers showed a high number of erythroblasts, suggesting extramedullary hematopoiesis in this organ as well. Pathological studies of livers revealed initial ballooning followed by progressive, age-dependent filling of sinusoidal cells and hepatocytes with vacuoles [10]. Skeletal abnormalities frequently occur in sialidosis II. According to researchers, a possible hypothesis explaining the underlying pathogenesis is the impaired function of osteoclasts resulting in inefficient bone remodeling and consequently leading to bone deformities [10]. Hearing loss is another feature of sialidosis II that appears late in the disease. Studies of the (KO)model showed both conductive and neurosensory defects contribute to hearing loss in *Neu1*−/− mice. It has been suggested that the absence of NEU1 and the potential exacerbation of lysosomal exocytosis in the inner ear are responsible for the occurrence of hearing the loss in *Neu1*−/− mice. Histopathological studies exhibited thickened, cerumen occlusion in the external auditory canal, while in the middle ear infiltration of connective tissue with signs of chronic inflammation was noticed. Also, in many cells of the extensive cochlea vacuolization was seen [56]. In the brain, *Neu1*-null mice show extensive vacuolization of the epithelial cells of the choroid plexus and the endothelial cells of the ependymal layer 31, 33. Microglia and perivascular macrophages were among the most affected cells. This feature was prominently noticeable in the dentate gyrus and the hippocampus, but these cells are also scattered throughout the cortex and in the cerebellum, causing a widespread microgliosis [10]. Additionally, in the hippocampal region of the *Neu1*-null mice, recent studies have suggested a link between NEU1 deficiency-exacerbated lysosomal exocytosis and the spontaneous occurrence of Alzheimer's disease (AD)-like amyloidogenic process. Essentially accumulation in endo-lysosomes of an over sialylated amyloid precursor protein (APP), which is a newly identified substrate of NEU1, initiates the process. Next Endo-lysosomal APP is proteolytically cleaved to generate amyloid β-peptide isoforms (Aβ), which is ultimately released extracellularly by excessive lysosomal exocytosis. The finding that intracranial injection of NEU1 in the AD mouse model reduces the numbers of amyloid plaques and the levels of amyloid peptides is exceptionally important, as it demonstrates that NEU1 can be explored as a therapeutic approach for AD [57].

Table 1. Clinical and Morphological findings of patients suffering from sialidosis II, congenital subtype form. (Cases from 1980 until present are included). M = male; F = female; n/a = not available; n/r = not reported; no = not detected.

References (Name of the First Author)	Gender	General Presentation	Nervous System	Ophthalmologic Findings	Skeleton	Respiratory Distress/Infections	Renal Involvement	Cardiac Involvement	Others	Course of Disease
Kelly, T.E. [23]	F	Ascites, edema, hepatosplenomegaly course features	n/r	n/r	Dysostosis multiplex	n/r	n/r	Cardiac anomalies	n/r	Exitus at 26 months
Riches, W.G. [24]	F	Hydrops, ascites, hepatosplenomegaly	n/r	n/r	n/r	n/r	n/r	n/r	n/r	Exitus at 4 months
Gillan, J.E. [25]	M	Hydrops, ascites, edema, hepatosplenomegaly course features	n/r	n/r	n/r	n/r	n/r	n/r	n/r	Exitus at 3 days
Beck, M. [26]	F	Hydrops, ascites, edema, hepato-splenomegaly, coarse features	n/r	n/r	n/r	present	present	n/r	n/r	Exitus at 6 months
Guibaud, P. [27]	F	Hydrops, ascites, edema, hepato-splenomegaly, coarse features	n/r	Corneal clouding	Dysostosis multiplex	n/r	n/r	n/r	n/r	n/r
Johnson, W.G. [28]	M M F F	Hydrops, Ascites, edema	Seizures	n/r	no	n/r	n/r	n/r	Telangiectasia	stillborn, 1 month, 3 months, alive 3 months
Yamano, T. [29]	M	Hydrops, ascites, edema, hepato-splenomegaly	n/a	no	no	n/a	n/a	n/a	n/a	Exitus at 56 days
Tabardel, Y. [30]	n/r	Hydrops, ascites, coarse features, hepatosplenomegaly	n/r	n/r	n/r	n/r	n/r	Cardiac anomalies	Petechiae	n/r
Ries, M. [31]	n/a	hydrops, ascites	n/r	Cherry red spots	n/r	n/r	n/r	n/r	n/r	Exitus at 28 days
Lukong, K.E. [9]	F	hydrops	n/r	n/r	n/r	n/r	n/r	n/r	n/r	Exitus at 82 days

Table 1. *Cont.*

References (Name of the First Author)	Gender	General Presentation	Nervous System	Ophthalmologic Findings	Skeleton	Respiratory Distress/Infections	Renal Involvement	Cardiac Involvement	Others	Course of Disease
Nakamura, Y. [32]	F	Ascites, coarse features, hepato-splenomegaly, inguinal hernia	Psychomotor retardation	n/r	Dysostosis multiplex	n/r	n/r	Cardiac anomalies	n/a	At the age of 2 months, patient was alive
Schmidt, M. [33]	F	Hydrops, ascites, edema, hepato-splenomegaly	Seizures	n/r	n/r	n/r	present	n/r	n/r	Exitus at 5 months
Ovali, F. [34]	M	Hydrops, ascites, coarse features, hepato-splenomegaly, inguinal hernia	n/r	n/r	n/r	n/r	present	n/r	n/r	Exitus at 27 days
Sergi, C. [35]	M	Hydrops, ascites, coarse features, hepato-splenomegaly, inguinal hernia	n/r	Corneal clouding	n/r	n/r	n/r	n/r	n/r	Exitus at 28 days
Sergi, C. [36]	M	Hydrops, edema ascites, hepato-splenomegaly	n/r	n/r	n/r	n/r	present	n/m/r	n/r	Exitus at 2 months
Buchholz, T. [37]	M	Hydrops, edema ascites, hepato-splenomegaly	n/a	n/a	n/a	present	n/a	Cardiac anomalies	Telangiectasia Hypotonia	Exitus at 82 days
Uhl, J. [38]	M M	Hydrops, edema, ascites in both patients	n/a	n/a	n/a	n/a	n/a	n/r	Polydactyly in patient 1	n/a
Donati, M.A. [39]	F	Hydrops, ascites, edema, coarse features, hepato-splenomegaly, Inguinal hernia	Psychomotor retardation, Hydrocephalus	yellow/rretina	Dysostosis multiplex	present	present	Cardiac anomalies	Telangiectasia Hypotonia, Petechiae	Exitus at 19 months
Penzel, R. [40]	F	Hydrops, ascites, edema	Seizures	n/r	n/r	n/r	n/r	n/r	n/r	n/r
Itoh, K. [41]	M	Hydrops, ascites, edema, hepato-splenomegaly	n/r	n/r	n/r	n/r	n/r	n/r	n/r	Exitus at 27 days

Table 1. *Cont.*

References (Name of the First Author)	Gender	General Presentation	Nervous System	Ophthalmologic Findings	Skeleton	Respiratory Distress/Infections	Renal Involvement	Cardiac Involvement	Others	Course of Disease
Rodriguez Criado, G. [12]	M	Hydrops, coarse features, hepatosplenomegaly	Psychomotor retardation	n/r	Dysostosis multiplex	n/r	n/r	Cardiac anomalies	Hypotonia	Exitus at 20 months
Pattison, S. [43]	n/r	n/r	n/r	n/r	n/r	n/r	n/r	n/r	n/r	Exitus at Patient 1; 3 months Patient 2; 2 months
Loren, D.J. [44]	n/r	Hydrops, ascites, edema, hepato-splenomegaly	n/r	n/r	no	n/r	n/r	n/r	n/r	Alive at the age of three months
Caciotti, A. [22]	F	Coarse features, hepatosplenomegaly	Psychomotor retardation	n/r	Dysostosis multiplex	n/r	present	Cardiac anomalies	Telangiectasia Hypotonia, petechiae	Exitus at 1 year
Bonten, E.J. [7]	F	Hydrops, hepato-splenomegaly	Psychomotor retardation, Hydrocephalus	No corneal opacity	Dysostosis multiplex, Joint contractures	n/r	n/r	cardiomyopathy	Cardiac anomalies	Exitus at 18 months
Lee, Y.J. [45]	F	Hydrops, ascites, coarse features, hepatosplenomegaly	n/r	Bilateral congenital cataracts with foveal hypoplasia	n/r	n/r	n/r	n/r	Telangiectasia Hypotonia, bluish to purpuric macules mild thrombocytopenia	Exitus a t9 months
Lee, B.H. [46]	F	Hydrops, ascites, coarse features, edema, hepato-splenomegaly	n/r	n/r	n/r	Present	n/r	Cardiomegaly with huge patent ductus arteriosus (PDA), Ventriculomegaly	Hypotonia	Exitus a t3 months

Table 2. Clinical and Morphological findings of patients suffering from sialidosis II, subtype infantile/Juvenile form (Cases from 1980 until the date of submission are included). M = male; F = female; n/a = not available n/r = not reported; no = not detected; ECG = electrocardiogram; ** Authors reported the case "suspected as sialidosis II" after other congenital errors of metabolism investigated during her childhood, such as mucopolysaccharidosis, were excluded. No formal genomic testing is reported in the study.

References (Name of the First Author)	Gender	General Presentation	Nervous System	Ophthalmologic Findings	Skeleton	Respiratory Distress/Infections	Renal Involvement	Cardiac Involvement	Others	Course of Disease
Winter, R.M. [47]	M <1 year	Coarse feature	Psychomotor delay, Seizures	Visual loss	Dysostosis Multiplex	n/r	n/r	n/r	Hearing loss, Inguinal hernia	22 years
Kelly, T.E. [23]	F <1 year	Coarse feature, Hepatosplenomegaly	Psychomotor delay, seizures/myoclonic jerks	Cherry red spot	Dysostosis Multiplex	present	n/r	present	Umbilical hernia	5 and half years
Kelly, T.E. [23]	F Birth	Coarse feature, Hepatosplenomegaly	Psychomotor delay	Cataract	Dysostosis Multiplex	n/r	n/r	present	Hearing loss, Umbilical hernia, Hypotonia	24 months
King, M. [48]	M 5 months	Coarse feature, Hepatosplenomegaly	Psychomotor delay Ataxia	Cherry red spot, corneal Clouding, Cataract,	Dysostosis Multiplex	n/r/	n/r	n/r	Hearing loss	13 years
King, M. [48]	F N/A	Coarse feature, Hepatosplenomegaly	Psychomotor delay	Cherry red spot, Cataract,	Dysostosis Multiplex	n/r	n/r	n/r	Hearing loss	12 years
Oohira, T. [49]	F <1 year	Coarse feature, Hepatosplenomegaly	Psychomotor delay, Ataxia, myoclonic jerks	Cherry red spots	Dysostosis Multiplex	n/r	n/r	n/r	Hypotonia	5 years
Young, I.D. [50]	M 18 months	Coarse feature	Psychomotor delay, Ataxia, myoclonic jerks	Cherry red spot, Nystagmus, Optic atrophy	Dysostosis Multiplex	nr	n/r	n/r	Hearing Loss, Hypotonia	12 years
Bakker, H.D. [51]	F 6 months	Coarse feature	Psychomotor delay	Strabismus, Nystagmus	n/r	n/r	n/r	n/r	Hearing Loss, Hypotonia	30 years
Rodriguez Criado, G. [42]	M <1 year	Coarse feature, Hepatosplenomegaly	Psychomotor delay, Myoclonic movements Ataxia	n/r	Dysostosis Multiplex	n/r	n/r	present	Hearing Loss, Hypotonia	13 years
Rodriguez Criado, G. [42]	M 16 months	Coarse feature, Hepatosplenomegaly	Psychomotor delay	n/r	Dysostosis Multiplex	n/r	n/r	absent	Hearing Loss, Hypotonia	11 years
Pattison, S. [43]	n/r	Coarse feature, Hepatosplenomegaly	n/r	n/r	Dysostosis Multiplex	n/r	n/r	n/r	n/r	3 years

Table 2. *Cont.*

References (Name of the First Author)	Gender	General Presentation	Nervous System	Ophthalmologic Findings	Skeleton	Respiratory Distress/Infections	Renal Involvement	Cardiac Involvement	Others	Course of Disease
Pattison, S. [43]	n/r	Coarse feature, Hepatosplenomegaly	n/r	n/r	Dysostosis Multiplex	n/r	n/r	n/r	n/r	3 years
Schiff, M. [52]	F <1 year	Coarse feature, Hepatosplenomegaly	Psychomotor delay	n/r	Dysostosis Multiplex	n/r	present	n/r	n/r	11 years
Gonzalez Gonzalez G [53]	n/r	n/r	Myoclonic epilepsy	n/r	Dysostosis Multiplex	n/r	n/r	present	n/r	14 years
Caciotti, A. [22]	M 1 year	Coarse feature	Psychomotor delay Seizures	Cherry red spot, cataract,	Dysostosis Multiplex	n/r	n/r	n/r	Hearing Loss	9 years
Bonten, E.J. [7]	M birth	Coarse feature, Hepatosplenomegaly	Developmental delay, Orbital hypoplasia	normal	Craniosynostosis	n/r	n/r	n/r	n/r	Progressing at 4 months
Bonten, E.J. [7]	F 12 years	n/r	Psychomotor delay, Seizures Ataxia, Dysmetria Spasticity	Cherry red spots	Dysostosis Multiplex, microcephaly	n/r	n/r	ECG specific alterations of repolarization	Hearing Loss1	Progressing at 28 years.
Ranganath, P [54]	F 18 months	Coarse facies, hepatomegaly	n/a	Mild corneal haziness, bilateral fundal Cherry red spots	Macrocephaly	n/r	n/r	Cardiac anomalies	Protuberant tongue, gum hypertrophy, generalized hypertrichosis, large Mongolian spots on the back, umbilical hernia	n/r
de Rezende Pintoi **[55]	F 30 years	a high forehead and low-set ears	Advanced degree of mental deficiency.lower limb spasticity, and facial and limb myoclonic jerks	Bilateral macular cherry-red spots	n/r	n/r	n/r	n/r	A marked delayed in motor and cognitive functions present since childhood. Cognitive and motor skills had worsened over 10 years	n/r

4. Therapeutic Interventions for Sialidosis

Due to the rarity of the disease, establishing optimum therapeutic measures remains a challenge although many promising methods are being proposed and being investigated. One attempt of enzyme replacement therapy (ERT) in *Neu1−/−* mice using a recombinant NEU1 enzyme purified from overexpressing insect cells was made, which helped significantly in increasing levels of the NEU1 protein, and this treatment achieved subsequent correction of the underlying pathology in most of the systemic organs. However, the recombinant protein turned out to be highly immunogenic in the mutant mice and thus causes a severe immune response. Consequently, the therapeutic use of ERT became restricted [58,59]. Another study investigated the efficacy of the immuno-suppressant (Celastrol) along with a proteasomal inhibitor (MG132) as a therapeutic option for sialidosis. Researchers found that MG132 enhances enzyme activity and its localization in cells expressing defective sialidase provided promising results [60]. Additionally, chaperone-mediated gene therapy using a new mouse model has been suggested. The new mouse model ubiquitously expresses a NEU1 variant, which has a V54M amino acid substitution found in an adult patient with type I sialidosis. Mutant mice exhibited signs of lysosomal disease after one year of age, with low residual NEU1 activity detected in most organs and cell types. Injection of aged mutant mice with AAV-PPCA caused improvement of symptoms in the disease phenotype, hence suggesting that some NEU1 mutations associated with type I sialidosis may respond to PPCA-chaperone-mediated gene therapy [61]. Researchers believe that the treatment may be useful for other NEU1 mutations, particularly those in patients with type I sialidosis [8].

5. Conclusions and Future Perspectives

Sialidosis is an autosomal recessive disease resulting due to a mutation in the neuraminidase (*NEU1*) gene. Missense mutations appear to be the most commonly occurring. Among these mutations, a significant molecular heterogeneity is present, with a mixed variety of clinical phenotypes presenting either as sialidosis I or sialidosis II with different levels of severity. The onset of disease, the severity of symptoms, and prognosis differ in sialidosis I and sialidosis II. Bonten et al. demonstrated that this association between the clinical phenotype and severity of the disease is the result of the residual activity of the mutant enzymes. Patients with type II disease have catalytic inactive neuraminidase, while patients with the mild type I disease have active catalytic neuraminidase. In the type I disease, there is an absence of any obvious physical defects, and life expectancy remains unaffected. However, progressive visual loss and myoclonus, which may tend to get worse with time, can be disabling. In type II, the congenital subtype takes a fulminant course with very low life expectancy. Ascites and edema are the prominent features of this subgroup of the disease. In the infantile/juvenile sub type, characteristic features include hepatosplenomegaly, dysostosis multiplex, coarse facies, cherry-red spot, myoclonus, and severe mental retardation. Some clinical manifestations such as ataxia and hearing loss may become progressively severe with age. In the last decade, atypical cases of sialidosis 1 have been reported, and this aspect warrants further studies in this area to investigate if there are more cases of sialidosis I than initially predicted. Furthermore, the possibility suggested by previous researchers that, in addition to neuraminidase mutations, environmental factors including diet, prophylactic therapies, or other genetic factors may have some effect on the penetrance and severity of the disease and/or phenotype of the disease seems more plausible [7]. Perhaps in the future, a more detailed prenatal history inquiring about the diet, medication, and different types of environmental exposure of parents may help the researchers understand this aspect of the disease. Therapeutic options for sialidosis remain limited. Researchers have emphasized exploring treatment options for sialidosis I [8]. In sialidosis I, symptoms are relatively mild and appear late. Although intelligence level remains normal, myoclonus can be debilitating. Therefore, effective therapy may improve quality of life. In sialidosis type II patients, an early onset, systemic involvement, and a fulminant course make it more challenging to provide treatment. Perhaps it would be worthwhile to explore the suggestion of taking an in utero approach for therapy in the future. Alternatively, carrier detection in affected families, prenatal molecular diagnosis, and improved genetic counseling seem to be a suitable practical approaches.

Finally, NEU1 appears to have a crucial link with the CNS. Studies provide substantial evidence to demonstrate the NEU1 enzyme has a correlation with Alzheimer's disease. Further understanding of NEU1 and its link with the CNS may provide useful information regarding genetics, pathogenesis, and treatment of not only sialidosis, but also Alzheimer's disease.

Conflicts of Interest: The authors declare no conflict of interest.

References

1. Pshezhetsky, A.V.; Richard, C.; Michaud, L.; Igdoura, S.; Wang, S.; Elsliger, M.A.; Qu, J.; Leclerc, D.; Gravel, R.; Dallaire, L.; et al. Cloning, expression and chromosomal mapping of human lysosomal sialidase and characterization of mutations in sialidosis. *Nat. Genet.* **1997**, *15*, 316–320. [CrossRef] [PubMed]

2. Bonten, E.; van der Spoel, A.; Fornerod, M.; Grosveld, G.; d'Azzo, A. Characterization of human lysosomal neuraminidase defines the molecular basis of the metabolic storage disorder sialidosis. *Genes Dev.* **1996**, *10*, 3156–3169. [CrossRef] [PubMed]

3. Cantz, M.; Gehler, J.; Spranger, J. Mucolipidosis I: Increased sialic acid content and deficiency of an alpha-n-acetylneuraminidase in cultured fibroblasts. *Biochem. Biophys. Res. Commun.* **1977**, *74*, 732–738. [CrossRef]

4. Sphranger, J.; Gehler, J.; Cantz, M. Mucolipidosis i—A sialidosis. *Am. J. Med. Genet.* **1977**, *1*, 21–29. [CrossRef] [PubMed]

5. Lowden, J.A.; O'Brien, J.S. Sialidosis: A review of human neuraminidase deficiency. *Am. J. Hum. Genet.* **1979**, *31*, 1–18. [PubMed]

6. Bonten, E.J.; Annunziata, I.; d'Azzo, A. Lysosomal multienzyme complex: Pros and cons of working together. *Cell. Mol. Life Sci.* **2014**, *71*, 2017–2032. [CrossRef] [PubMed]

7. Bonten, E.J.; Arts, W.F.; Beck, M.; Covanis, A.; Donati, M.A.; Parini, R.; Zammarchi, E.; d'Azzo, A. Novel mutations in lysosomal neuraminidase identify functional domains and determine clinical severity in sialidosis. *Hum. Mol. Genet.* **2000**, *9*, 2715–2725. [CrossRef] [PubMed]

8. D'Azzo, A.; Machado, E.; Annunziata, I. Pathogenesis, emerging therapeutic targets and treatment in sialidosis. *Expert Opin. Orphan Drugs* **2015**, *3*, 491–504. [CrossRef] [PubMed]

9. Lukong, K.E.; Elsliger, M.A.; Chang, Y.; Richard, C.; Thomas, G.; Carey, W.; Tylki-Szymanska, A.; Czartoryska, B.; Buchholz, T.; Criado, G.R.; et al. Characterization of the sialidase molecular defects in sialidosis patients suggests the structural organization of the lysosomal multienzyme complex. *Hum. Mol. Genet.* **2000**, *9*, 1075–1085. [CrossRef] [PubMed]

10. De Geest, N.; Bonten, E.; Mann, L.; de Sousa-Hitzler, J.; Hahn, C.; d'Azzo, A. Systemic and neurologic abnormalities distinguish the lysosomal disorders sialidosis and galactosialidosis in mice. *Hum. Mol. Genet.* **2002**, *11*, 1455–1464. [CrossRef] [PubMed]

11. Yogalingam, G.; Bonten, E.J.; van de Vlekkert, D.; Hu, H.; Moshiach, S.; Connell, S.A.; d'Azzo, A. Neuraminidase 1 is a negative regulator of lysosomal exocytosis. *Dev. Cell* **2008**, *15*, 74–86. [CrossRef] [PubMed]

12. Dridi, L.; Seyrantepe, V.; Fougerat, A.; Pan, X.; Bonneil, E.; Thibault, P.; Moreau, A.; Mitchell, G.A.; Heveker, N.; Cairo, C.W.; et al. Positive regulation of insulin signaling by neuraminidase 1. *Diabetes* **2013**, *62*, 2338–2346. [CrossRef] [PubMed]

13. Sobral, I.; Cachulo Mda, L.; Figueira, J.; Silva, R. Sialidosis type i: Ophthalmological findings. *BMJ Case Rep.* **2014**, *2014*. [CrossRef] [PubMed]

14. Franceschetti, S.; Canafoglia, L. Sialidoses. *Epileptic Disord.* **2016**, *18*, 89–93. [PubMed]

15. Takahashi, Y.; Nakamura, Y.; Yamaguchi, S.; Orii, T. Urinary oligosaccharide excretion and severity of galactosialidosis and sialidosis. *Clin. Chim. Acta* **1991**, *203*, 199–210. [CrossRef]

16. Sekijima, Y.; Nakamura, K.; Kishida, D.; Narita, A.; Adachi, K.; Ohno, K.; Nanba, E.; Ikeda, S. Clinical and serial mri findings of a sialidosis type i patient with a novel missense mutation in the neu1 gene. *Intern. Med.* **2013**, *52*, 119–124. [CrossRef] [PubMed]

17. Huang, Y.Z.; Lai, S.C.; Lu, C.S.; Weng, Y.H.; Chuang, W.L.; Chen, R.S. Abnormal cortical excitability with preserved brainstem and spinal reflexes in sialidosis type i. *Clin. Neurophysiol.* **2008**, *119*, 1042–1050. [CrossRef] [PubMed]

18. Palmeri, S.; Villanova, M.; Malandrini, A.; van Diggelen, O.P.; Huijmans, J.G.; Ceuterick, C.; Rufa, A.; DeFalco, D.; Ciacci, G.; Martin, J.J.; et al. Type i sialidosis: A clinical, biochemical and neuroradiological study. *Eur. Neurol.* **2000**, *43*, 88–94. [CrossRef] [PubMed]

19. Thomas, G.H.; Tipton, R.E.; Ch'ien, L.T.; Reynolds, L.W.; Miller, C.S. Sialidase (alpha-n-acetyl neuraminidase) deficiency: The enzyme defect in an adult with macular cherry-red spots and myoclonus without dementia. *Clin. Genet.* **1978**, *13*, 369–379. [CrossRef] [PubMed]

20. Franceschetti, S.; Uziel, G.; Di Donato, S.; Caimi, L.; Avanzini, G. Cherry-red spot myoclonus syndrome and alpha-neuraminidase deficiency: Neurophysiological, pharmacological and biochemical study in an adult. *J. Neurol. Neurosurg. Psychiatry* **1980**, *43*, 934–940. [CrossRef] [PubMed]

21. Canafoglia, L.; Robbiano, A.; Pareyson, D.; Panzica, F.; Nanetti, L.; Giovagnoli, A.R.; Venerando, A.; Gellera, C.; Franceschetti, S.; Zara, F. Expanding sialidosis spectrum by genome-wide screening: Neu1 mutations in adult-onset myoclonus. *Neurology* **2014**, *82*, 2003–2006. [CrossRef] [PubMed]

22. Caciotti, A.; Di Rocco, M.; Filocamo, M.; Grossi, S.; Traverso, F.; d'Azzo, A.; Cavicchi, C.; Messeri, A.; Guerrini, R.; Zammarchi, E.; et al. Type ii sialidosis: Review of the clinical spectrum and identification of a new splicing defect with chitotriosidase assessment in two patients. *J. Neurol.* **2009**, *256*, 1911–1915. [CrossRef] [PubMed]

23. Kelly, T.E.; Bartoshesky, L.; Harris, D.J.; McCauley, R.G.; Feingold, M.; Schott, G. Mucolipidosis i (acid neuraminidase deficiency). Three cases and delineation of the variability of the phenotype. *Am. J. Dis. Child.* **1981**, *135*, 703–708. [CrossRef] [PubMed]

24. Riches, W.G.; Smuckler, E.A. A severe infantile mucolipidosis. Clinical, biochemical, and pathologic features. *Arch. Pathol. Lab. Med.* **1983**, *107*, 147–152. [PubMed]

25. Gillan, J.E.; Lowden, J.A.; Gaskin, K.; Cutz, E. Congenital ascites as a presenting sign of lysosomal storage disease. *J. Pediatr.* **1984**, *104*, 225–231. [CrossRef]

26. Beck, M.; Bender, S.W.; Reiter, H.L.; Otto, W.; Bassler, R.; Dancygier, H.; Gehler, J. Neuraminidase deficiency presenting as non-immune hydrops fetalis. *Eur. J. Pediatr.* **1984**, *143*, 135–139. [CrossRef] [PubMed]

27. Guibaud, P.; Cottin, X.; Maire, I.; Boyer, S.; Guibaud, S.; Coicaud, C.; Bellon-Azzouzi, C.; Duvernois, J.P. fetal ascites as a manifestation of infantile sialidosis. Significance of a study of oligosaccharides in amniotic fluid. *J. Genet. Hum.* **1985**, *33*, 317–324. [PubMed]

28. Johnson, W.G.; Thomas, G.H.; Miranda, A.F.; Driscoll, J.M.; Wigger, J.H.; Yeh, M.N.; Schwartz, R.C.; Cohen, C.S.; Berdon, W.E.; Koenigsberger, M.R. Congenital sialidosis: Biochemical studies: Clinical spectrum in four sibs; two successful prenatal diagnoses (abstract). *Am. J. Hum. Genet.* **1980**, *32*, A43.

29. Yamano, T.; Shimada, M.; Matsuzaki, K.; Matsumoto, Y.; Yoshihara, W.; Okada, S.; Inui, K.; Yutaka, T.; Yabuuchi, H. Pathological study on a severe sialidosis (alpha-neuraminidase deficiency). *Acta Neuropathol.* **1986**, *71*, 278–284. [CrossRef] [PubMed]

30. Tabardel, Y.; Soyeur, D.; Vivario, E.; Senterre, J. primary neuraminidase deficiency with prenatal disclosure. *Arch. Fr. Pediatr.* **1989**, *46*, 737–740. [PubMed]

31. Ries, M.; Deeg, K.H.; Wolfel, D.; Ibel, H.; Maier, B.; Buheitel, G. Colour doppler imaging of intracranial vasculopathy in severe infantile sialidosis. *Pediatr. Radiol.* **1992**, *22*, 179–181. [CrossRef] [PubMed]

32. Nakamura, Y.; Takahashi, Y.; Yamaguchi, S.; Omiya, S.; Orii, T.; Yara, A.; Gushiken, M. Severe infantile sialidosis—The characteristics of oligosaccharides isolated from the urine and the abdominal ascites. *Tohoku J. Exp. Med.* **1992**, *166*, 407–415. [CrossRef] [PubMed]

33. Schmidt, M.; Fahnenstich, H.; Haverkamp, F.; Platz, H.; Hansmann, M.; Bartmann, P. sialidosis and galactosialidosis as the cause of non-immunologic hydrops fetalis. *Z Geburtshilfe Neonatol.* **1997**, *201*, 177–180. [PubMed]

34. Ovali, F.; Samanci, N.; Guray, A.; Akdogan, Z.; Akdeniz, C.; Dagoglu, T.; Petorak, I. Congenital sialidosis. *Turk. J. Pediatr.* **1998**, *40*, 447–451. [PubMed]

35. Sergi, C.; Beedgen, B.; Kopitz, J.; Zilow, E.; Zoubaa, S.; Otto, H.F.; Cantz, M.; Linderkamp, O. Refractory congenital ascites as a manifestation of neonatal sialidosis: Clinical, biochemical and morphological studies in a newborn syrian male infant. *Am. J. Perinatol.* **1999**, *16*, 133–141. [CrossRef] [PubMed]

36. Sergi, C.; Penzel, R.; Uhl, J.; Zoubaa, S.; Dietrich, H.; Decker, N.; Rieger, P.; Kopitz, J.; Otto, H.F.; Kiessling, M.; et al. Prenatal diagnosis and fetal pathology in a turkish family harboring a novel nonsense mutation in the lysosomal alpha-n-acetyl-neuraminidase (sialidase) gene. *Hum. Genet.* **2001**, *109*, 421–428. [CrossRef] [PubMed]

37. Buchholz, T.; Molitor, G.; Lukong, K.E.; Praun, M.; Genzel-Boroviczeny, O.; Freund, M.; Pshezhetsky, A.V.; Schulze, A. Clinical presentation of congenital sialidosis in a patient with a neuraminidase gene frameshift mutation. *Eur. J. Pediatr.* **2001**, *160*, 26–30. [CrossRef] [PubMed]

38. Uhl, J.; Penzel, R.; Sergi, C.; Kopitz, J.; Otto, H.F.; Cantz, M. Identification of a ctl4/neu1 fusion transcript in a sialidosis patient. *FEBS Lett.* **2002**, *521*, 19–23. [CrossRef]

39. Donati, M.A.; Caciotti, A.; Bardelli, T.; Dani, C.; d'Azzo, A.; Morrone, A.; Zammarchi, E. Congenital sialidosis hydrops fetalis neuraminidase hydrocephalus sialidosis congenita idrope fetale neuraminidase idrocefalo. *Ital. J. Pediatr.* **2003**, *29*, 404–410.

40. Penzel, R.; Uhl, J.; Kopitz, J.; Beck, M.; Otto, H.F.; Cantz, M. Splice donor site mutation in the lysosomal neuraminidase gene causing exon skipping and complete loss of enzyme activity in a sialidosis patient. *FEBS Lett.* **2001**, *501*, 135–138. [CrossRef]

41. Itoh, K.; Naganawa, Y.; Matsuzawa, F.; Aikawa, S.; Doi, H.; Sasagasako, N.; Yamada, T.; Kira, J.; Kobayashi, T.; Pshezhetsky, A.V.; et al. Novel missense mutations in the human lysosomal sialidase gene in sialidosis patients and prediction of structural alterations of mutant enzymes. *J. Hum. Genet.* **2002**, *47*, 29–37. [CrossRef] [PubMed]

42. Rodriguez Criado, G.; Pshezhetsky, A.V.; Rodriguez Becerra, A.; Gomez de Terreros, I. Clinical variability of type ii sialidosis by c808t mutation. *Am. J. Med. Genet. A* **2003**, *116A*, 368–371. [CrossRef] [PubMed]

43. Pattison, S.; Pankarican, M.; Rupar, C.A.; Graham, F.L.; Igdoura, S.A. Five novel mutations in the lysosomal sialidase gene (neu1) in type ii sialidosis patients and assessment of their impact on enzyme activity and intracellular targeting using adenovirus-mediated expression. *Hum. Mutat.* **2004**, *23*, 32–39. [CrossRef] [PubMed]

44. Loren, D.J.; Campos, Y.; d'Azzo, A.; Wyble, L.; Grange, D.K.; Gilbert-Barness, E.; White, F.V.; Hamvas, A. Sialidosis presenting as severe nonimmune fetal hydrops is associated with two novel mutations in lysosomal alpha-neuraminidase. *J. Perinatol.* **2005**, *25*, 491–494. [CrossRef] [PubMed]

45. Lee, Y.J.; Son, S.K.; Park, J.H.; Song, J.S.; Cheon, C.K. Neu1 mutation in a korean infant with type 2 sialidosis presenting as isolated fetal ascites. *Pediatr. Neonatol.* **2015**, *56*, 68–69. [CrossRef] [PubMed]

46. Lee, B.H.; Kim, Y.M.; Kim, J.H.; Kim, G.H.; Lee, B.S.; Kim, C.J.; Yoo, H.J.; Yoo, H.W. Histological, biochemical, and genetic characterization of early-onset fulminating sialidosis type 2 in a korean neonate with hydrops fetalis. *Brain Dev.* **2014**, *36*, 171–175. [CrossRef] [PubMed]

47. Winter, R.M.; Swallow, D.M.; Baraitser, M.; Purkiss, P. Sialidosis type 2 (acid neuraminidase deficiency): Clinical and biochemical features of a further case. *Clin. Genet.* **1980**, *18*, 203–210. [CrossRef] [PubMed]

48. King, M.; Cockburn, F.; MacPhee, G.B.; Logan, R.W. Infantile type 2 sialidosis in a pakistani family—A clinical and biochemical study. *J. Inherit. Metab. Dis.* **1984**, *7*, 91–96. [CrossRef] [PubMed]

49. Oohira, T.; Nagata, N.; Akaboshi, I.; Matsuda, I.; Naito, S. The infantile form of sialidosis type ii associated with congenital adrenal hyperplasia: Possible linkage between hla and the neuraminidase deficiency gene. *Hum. Genet.* **1985**, *70*, 341–343. [CrossRef] [PubMed]

50. Young, I.D.; Young, E.P.; Mossman, J.; Fielder, A.R.; Moore, J.R. Neuraminidase deficiency: Case report and review of the phenotype. *J. Med. Genet.* **1987**, *24*, 283–290. [CrossRef] [PubMed]

51. Bakker, H.D.; Abeling, N.G.G.M.; Staalman, C.R.; van Gennip, A.H. Thirty-years follow-up of a patient with sialidosis. *J. Inherit. Metab. Dis.* **1998**, *21*, 116.

52. Schiff, M.; Maire, I.; Bertrand, Y.; Cochat, P.; Guffon, N. Long-term follow-up of metachronous marrow-kidney transplantation in severe type ii sialidosis: What does success mean? *Nephrol. Dial. Transplant.* **2005**, *20*, 2563–2565. [CrossRef] [PubMed]

53. Gonzalez Gonzalez, G.; Jimenez Lopez, I. anesthetic management of a boy with sialidosis. *Rev. Esp. Anestesiol. Reanim.* **2006**, *53*, 253–256. [PubMed]

54. Ranganath, P.; Sharma, V.; Danda, S.; Nandineni, M.R.; Dalal, A.B. Novel mutations in the neuraminidase-1 (neu1) gene in two patients of sialidosis in india. *Indian J. Med. Res.* **2012**, *136*, 1048–1050. [PubMed]

55. Vieira de Rezende Pinto, W.B.; Sgobbi de Souza, P.V.; Pedroso, J.L.; Barsottini, O.G. Variable phenotype and severity of sialidosis expressed in two siblings presenting with ataxia and macular cherry-red spots. *J. Clin. Neurosci.* **2013**, *20*, 1327–1328. [CrossRef] [PubMed]

56. Wu, X.; Steigelman, K.A.; Bonten, E.; Hu, H.; He, W.; Ren, T.; Zuo, J.; d'Azzo, A. Vacuolization and alterations of lysosomal membrane proteins in cochlear marginal cells contribute to hearing loss in neuraminidase 1-deficient mice. *Biochim. Biophys. Acta* **2010**, *1802*, 259–268. [CrossRef] [PubMed]

57. Annunziata, I.; Patterson, A.; Helton, D.; Hu, H.; Moshiach, S.; Gomero, E.; Nixon, R.; d'Azzo, A. Lysosomal NEU1 deficiency affects amyloid precursor protein levels and amyloid-β secretion via deregulated lysosomal exocytosis. *Nat. Commun.* **2013**, *4*, 2734. [CrossRef] [PubMed]

58. Bonten, E.J.; Wang, D.; Toy, J.N.; Mann, L.; Mignardot, A.; Yogalingam, G.; D'Azzo, A. Targeting macrophages with baculovirus-produced lysosomal enzymes: Implications for enzyme replacement therapy of the glycoprotein storage disorder galactosialidosis. *FASEB J.* **2004**, *18*, 971–973. [CrossRef] [PubMed]

59. Wang, D.; Bonten, E.J.; Yogalingam, G.; Mann, L.; d'Azzo, A. Short-term, high dose enzyme replacement therapy in sialidosis mice. *Mol. Genet. Metab.* **2005**, *85*, 181–189. [CrossRef] [PubMed]

60. O'Leary, E.M.; Igdoura, S.A. The therapeutic potential of pharmacological chaperones and proteosomal inhibitors, celastrol and mg132 in the treatment of sialidosis. *Mol. Genet. Metab.* **2012**, *107*, 173–185. [CrossRef] [PubMed]

61. Bonten, E.J.; Yogalingam, G.; Hu, H.; Gomero, E.; van de Vlekkert, D.; d'Azzo, A. Chaperone-mediated gene therapy with recombinant aav-ppca in a new mouse model of type i sialidosis. *Biochim. Biophys. Acta* **2013**, *1832*, 1784–1792. [CrossRef] [PubMed]

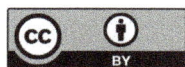

MDPI

St. Alban-Anlage 66

4052 Basel

Switzerland

Tel. +41 61 683 77 34

Fax +41 61 302 89 18

www.mdpi.com

Diagnostics Editorial Office

E-mail: diagnostics@mdpi.com

www.mdpi.com/journal/diagnostics

www.ingramcontent.com/pod-product-compliance
Lightning Source LLC
Chambersburg PA
CBHW051908210326
41597CB00033B/6071